Commissioning and a Population Approach to Health Services Decision-Making

Commissioning and a Population Approach to Health Services Decision-Making

Julie Sin, MB ChB, DCH, MRCGP, MFPHM, FFPH

*Fellow of the Faculty of Public Health, formerly Governing Body Member,
NHS Eastern Cheshire Clinical Commissioning Group, and Consultant
in Public Health Medicine, Cheshire East Unitary Authority, UK*

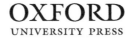

OXFORD
UNIVERSITY PRESS

OXFORD
UNIVERSITY PRESS

Great Clarendon Street, Oxford, OX2 6DP,
United Kingdom

Oxford University Press is a department of the University of Oxford.
It furthers the University's objective of excellence in research, scholarship,
and education by publishing worldwide. Oxford is a registered trade mark of
Oxford University Press in the UK and in certain other countries

Published in the United States of America by Oxford University Press
198 Madison Avenue, New York, NY 10016, United States of America

British Library Cataloguing in Publication Data

Data available

Library of Congress Control Number: 2020942405
ISBN 978–0–19–884073–2

Printed in Great Britain by
Ashford Colour Press Ltd, Gosport, Hampshire

For Isabella and Louis

Preface

If you had asked me when I started in the health service what I would be talking about now, I would not have said commissioning. Child health, elderly care, general practice, or psychiatry perhaps, something connected with people I would have thought. I probably would have asked what commissioning was which would have been quite a reasonable question 30 years ago. Since then, this layer of work to plan, secure, and make decisions about health services for populations has not stood still within health services in England, and there have been several iterations of how commissioning has been organized in that time. And yes it ultimately concerns people.

In recent years there has been an increasing emphasis on a population perspective to commissioning and health services decision-making. This involves building and enabling a system to do this and this requires a mindset with population concepts at its core. Experience of working with practitioners in commissioning (from many backgrounds) and those training for practice is that whilst the importance of ideas may be grasped, they might still be left ill-prepared to incorporate these ideas into practice. This book offers a contribution as to how this might be done.

This book is based on over 20 years of working in the commissioning arena across strategic, local, and collaborative footprints, and also draws from a wide clinical and population health experience alongside that. Over this time it has been loud and clear that a population perspective is absolutely integral to all of commissioning. This was not just about technical inputs to produce a thing for this or for that, it was also about the practical use of knowledge and the thinking processes behind the decisions that resulted from the so-called processes of commissioning.

After over two decades of working in the health services commissioning arena in its various guises, it is still striking how the underpinning concepts of a population approach are consistent whatever the behind-the-scenes NHS structures of the day. Over this time I have had the humbling experience of seeing different commissioning formats come and go; of seeing close up the system context from strategic, local, and collaborative perspectives; and I have worked with colleagues of many backgrounds, all contributing to the commissioning effort and all trying to make sense of the same basic issue of achieving health gain with finite resources in a commissioning system. What is clear is that the core bearings to help do this are always useful whatever the commissioning formats of the day. In this book I have therefore gathered together the key concepts and approaches that have been perennially helpful over this time, in one place, in case useful for others too.

This book is written for people who want to learn about commissioning and taking a population approach to health services decision-making, whether or not they are taking a course in it.

From experience of working in the commissioning arena, one of the challenges is that colleagues are often expected to operate effectively in many applied scenarios (for example with the prioritization of resources, collaborative commissioning, or whole-system strategy scenario) without sufficient orientation about the core themes of commissioning for populations. They may struggle in that setting not from lack of managerial competence but from lack of practical orientation. This book is intended to help.

I wanted to create a book containing key pointers to the topic all in one place and written from a commissioning perspective. One that acknowledges that it can be messy in real life but there are 'thought journeys' that can help work through practical alternatives and handling of such commissioning challenges. I wanted a book to help improve understanding of common language to think about health gain and the systems and levers to achieve that, and a book that would be useful whatever the structural system of the day, because issues of finite resources, securing quality health services, and reducing health inequalities will always be pertinent.

At many points of putting this together, it has of course felt like standing on the shoulders of giants, past and present, to be able to see the view from a commissioning angle. For that I am very grateful and hope I can help introduce the messages to some new people. I am grateful also for the wisdom and support of the UK Specialised Commissioning Public Health Network (later the UK Commissioning Public Health Network), especially during the years when commissioning seemed to be defined as the sum of different streams of spending and spenders rather than for its population health purpose. For the real life learning through our trials and tribulations to achieve the best we can with the resources in hand, I thank the many colleagues at the coal face of commissioning and public health over the years in the many different settings; the learning has helped to ground this book. I am also grateful to the people and carers that make up the populations that commissioned services are intended to be there for, for being a sentinel reminder of why taking a population approach to commissioning is so important. Thank you too to my family for their enduring support and encouraging me whilst I put this together.

Chapters can be taken as individual portions if preferred, or taken as a whole. I hope this offering of pointers and insights helps to complement your repertoire of skills, whatever your starting point with commissioning.

Contents

PART II: ENABLING LEADERSHIP FOR A POPULATION APPROACH TO HEALTH SERVICES DECISION-MAKING

PART I

CORE CONCEPTS FOR A POPULATION APPROACH TO HEALTH SERVICES DECISION-MAKING

1

Introduction

Imagine a world where there's a new problem to be solved. Imagine that a new bunch of people have been brought together to solve it. Imagine that lives depended on their efforts. There has been little formal training for this particular situation and many of the old familiar faces and structures have recently changed. If they were to be honest, few could truly say they were confident that they knew what they were doing. What they did know was that they had an important job to do, that they were caretakers of a certain amount of money, and that other people's lives could be at stake. Since no one is completely sure what the best way of tackling the problem is, they decide to organize themselves into a hierarchy to create a sense of order. Soon they are organized and they have a means of command and control. However, getting to grips with how to address the problem remains elusive. The group continues to do its best but always wonders if it could be a bit easier, a bit clearer, and a bit less stressful.

Now imagine a world where everyone involved feels they have sufficient confidence and competence to contribute in a meaningful way. There is good understanding of the issues and everything that is done is aimed at chipping away at the problem to be solved either directly or indirectly. If any actions turned out not to be effective they would be stopped. There is still some central control but it manages to encourage effective contributions. Everyone is confident to try, and learn from their experiences to do their best for now and hopefully be even more effective in the future. They are aware that it is not always easy but they know their efforts have a good chance of going somewhere and are resilient enough to deal with many new changes in the external landscape.

This book is about moving closer to this second position in thinking about health services and commissioning for populations. In particular it is about commissioning and health services decision-making for better population health outcomes.

In the arena of healthcare commissioning, decision-making is about how best to address health needs and improve population outcomes with the resources available in a real-life context: that is the challenge. Commissioning

Commissioning and a Population Approach to Health Services Decision-Making. Julie Sin, Oxford University Press (2020). © Oxford University Press. DOI: 10.1093/oso/9780198840732.001.0001

is the term given to encompass the collection of processes to help with that challenge. This often takes place in a context of incomplete information and timescale constraints as well as limited resources. So how can one commission effectively with better population outcomes in mind? Some bearings and tools to help find a way through and make sense of things would be useful.

The book is written with the busy practitioner in mind and is intended to be of use whether you work in this area regularly, or perhaps you have specific expertise in another area but have been called upon to take part in bigger population-wide decisions, or you just need a big picture understanding of the healthcare system. From the outset it is intended to help with day to day or strategic decision-making, by unlocking situations and helping to set off on the right track.

It is to help colleagues working in health services commissioning at all levels of contribution (whether working on day to day processes or board level); public health professionals working in the quality and commissioning arena; and all students and 'trainees' in the pipeline whose future work might involve commissioning services or healthcare public health. Those who work with commissioners of health services may also find the topics useful.

The book is an armoury of key concepts or 'navigation tools' to help with decision-making for better population outcomes whatever your role is within commissioning in the health system. It brings together a range of essential perspectives in one place to help understand context, purpose, and levers in the system for better strategic discussions and decision-making. If you are new to services commissioning and find yourself here, I hope it helps you with an accelerated start to your healthcare system journey. For those who may be more familiar with the commissioning landscape I hope you find this collection of vantage points in one place helpful for practice and also for helping others with this territory.

It will take you through the fundamental concepts needed for commissioning for a population. It assumes no expert knowledge on commissioning, just an inclination to become familiar with ideas to enhance the population perspective to health services decision-making.

The longer view

The 'evolution' of health services is likely to continue but the basic challenge in aiming for population health gain with finite resources will remain as long as health services coverage is for whole populations. Indeed at times of change, the population bearings in the book become even more relevant in helping to focus on the health outcomes despite structural changes, and the book may help a new generation of colleagues as necessary. For example, the further development of integrated models of care delivery such as that of primary care services with other community care providers; or across primary care and specialist care providers; or even more integrated models will still involve the perennial considerations of how best to achieve population health gain with finite resources. Whether these population level considerations will continue to be borne by commissioning organizations ('commissioners') alone or be increasingly shared between commissioners and providers, only time will tell.

What the book is about

Essentially, the health service commissioning machinery needs a population perspective to help it achieve better population outcomes from available resources. The book focuses on this important link and the practical knowledge and concepts needed for working in this area.

After taking stock of what commissioning is in practice, and the crucial synergy needed between commissioning processes and population health gain, the chapters present key vantage points and further applied topics for commissioners.

The vantage points taken to help unlock this in practice can be applied to assist with the many questions that will invariably come up in commissioning situations. For example, what information is relevant? What can be done? What works best? What is going on? What is our role in this? These 'navigation tools' are intended to help you find your way through to making sense of the situation.

The book respects that real-life starting points are often not where you would ideally want them. However, you can still navigate your way towards better population outcomes making better use of healthcare resources regardless of where you start. Through surveying the opportunities, assessing which are more effective, prioritizing your resources, recognizing who your partners are and when to work closely and when to work loosely with them, you can raise the chances of better outcomes through your efforts. Issues are tackled from the perspective of someone working in the real-life commissioning scenario rather than from a purely theoretical perspective, though there is of course theoretical grounding throughout as applicable. It is a guide for the real life decision-maker who needs a conceptually robust, 'good enough' approach to do their everyday work of securing health services for the population they serve.

Unfortunately, commissioning robots as such do not exist and commissioning is the result of the combined efforts of all those working to secure services for their populations. It may comprise one hundred percent of someone's role, or just part of their role. As a set of skills and practical understanding, commissioning is an interdisciplinary endeavour. It is relevant to a wide range of people who might find themselves intentionally or 'accidently' contributing to the planning and securing of services for their populations. As one would expect in this interdisciplinary area, a degree of 'multilingualism' across professionals is helpful on occasions to appreciate the different contributions that colleagues bring to the table in health services decision-making for populations, and I hope the book brings a little of that too.

Setting and scope

The book is grounded in the experience of health services in England where at its core there is provision of a comprehensive range of health services on a whole population basis, free at the point of need. The underpinning concepts will be relevant to the reader as long as health services retain a population-wide scope. The reader is taken through the book using the main anchoring point of commissioning, the process of securing services for a population within finite resources. Concepts are covered with recognition of the contextual challenges of finite resources and the constant system evolution of health services that the practitioner has to operate in.

For expediency, the term 'health services' will be used in the book to encompass the range of services experienced by citizens as part of a population-wide health and healthcare provision. In 'current speak', this encompasses services that are presently administratively referred to as 'NHS commissioned' or 'Public Health commissioned' services. In general of course, the core commissioning concepts could also be applied to those aspects of social care commissioning which are organized on a population basis. Where the term 'health and care services' is used, it refers to the combination of health and social care services that are amenable to commissioning on a population basis. In this sense, the book's concepts are pertinent whatever one's local scope of health services or health and care services commissioning, as long as services are commissioned on a population basis. To many citizens of course, services are not differentiated by how the money flows behind the scenes (via various 'commissioners'), it is the coherence of the whole pathway that is important, and the scope of this book supports that aim.

How the book is structured

All chapters can be used as standalone items or can be taken as part of a whole collection. Each chapter covers an orientating concept (or a set of related concepts) that is pertinent to commissioning for populations. Each concept or vantage point is described and explained, and the connections to commissioning practice are discerned with practical reflections on their use. The book is presented in two parts. Part I contains core concepts needed for commissioning and health services decision-making, and offers concepts that tangibly link commissioning actions with a population approach. Part II contains the more applied topics and scenarios that commissioners will need to navigate in practice.

In the first half of the book (Part I), Chapter 2 provides orientation about the visible and behind-the-scenes components of a health system that plans, buys, and delivers care. Chapter 3 then looks at the logical overlap between a population view and commissioning and introduces core concepts for a population approach.

Chapter 4 is about the notional 'commissioning cycle' and the main activities it refers to. Chapter 5 invites the reader to be orientated to the terminology and practice of the public health specialty as this gives more insight into its overlaps with health services for populations in general.

Chapter 6 helps to make more sense of the evidence that you will come across in practice and facilitates understanding that some methods of gathering evidence of what works are more robust than others.

Chapter 7 invites the reader to look at commissioning through the lens of effective preventive opportunities, while Chapter 8 concludes the core orientation with a spotlight on using health information purposefully for commissioning. As with the first half, topics in Part II can be used as standalone items but also contribute to the overall coherence of the collection. Chapter 9 demonstrates that a population approach to decision-making and planning applies across strategic and operational levels of commissioning activity.

Chapter 10 concerns priority setting and having a coherent approach to decision-making. Chapter 11 looks at commissioning collaboratively and when that is sensible and when it is less so. Chapter 12 helps to recognize when you are dealing with a simple, complicated, or complex scenario, and to adjust your approach accordingly. Chapter 13 is an orientation to the basic dimensions of quality and a pragmatic look at quality from the commissioning perspective so you can make sense of the arena when doing this work. Chapter 14 looks at the role of commissioners in addressing health inequalities of access and outcomes of services. Chapter 15 will then bring us to the end of the navigation system for a population approach to commissioning, to reflect on where this has taken us, and hopefully to the start of many onward journeys using a population approach to health service decision-making.

The bearings offered in this book are designed to be useful whatever the style or structure of the day of the healthcare system. External changes might make you have to work differently (and the challenge then is to get to an equilibrium quickly), but the 'what to aim for' remains remarkably consistent as long as there is a whole population basis to secure services for. I hope you enjoy using this book.

2
Health System

Basic Structures

Before embarking on a journey into the world of health service commissioning, it is useful to know a little of the anatomy and workings of the territory we are about to enter. Just as one might have a pocket map of the main sights to help to get around a new city and to make quicker sense of what you see around you, it is useful to know some basic structures around the health system. You could of course just set off and there is nothing wrong with that, though it depends on your needs and starting point. In practice you may already have familiarity with an aspect, or several aspects, of the health system, perhaps through directly working in those areas, or have experience through another sector, or through experiences as a patient or carer.

This chapter will describe the main 'visible' and 'behind-the-scenes' components of the publicly funded English health service. Visible structures are the more tangible components of health services and are the more familiar aspects that the general population would easily recognize as health services. Access to these parts is either through direct access or via referral. Behind-the-scenes components are those aspects responsible for ensuring services are planned and acquired for the population served. This layer involves decisions about how resources are deployed to provide services delivered by the visible structures.

In England the term health service is largely synonymous with the National Health Service (NHS) and is often used interchangeably. It is important however to note that depending on the arrangements of the time, the scope of publicly funded health services can be wider than the services commissioned under the NHS umbrella alone (though the latter would be responsible for commissioning the vast bulk of health services free at the point of delivery). Over time there have been a range of publicly funded health services that are organized through local authorities (such as health visiting and immunizations in pre-1974 arrangements, and school nursing and sexual health services in the post-2013 arrangements).[1,2] Such services

Commissioning and a Population Approach to Health Services Decision-Making. Julie Sin, Oxford University Press (2020). © Oxford University Press. DOI: 10.1093/oso/9780198840732.001.0001

are also part of the entirety of health services experienced by the population. For that reason the term health services will be used in general to refer to the publicly funded health services as a whole, where the funds originate from national government allocation. Where it is more useful to the use the term the National Health Service, for example when it has a specific administrative definition, the term NHS will be used.

The 'visible' components

There is a range of visible components to provide care as part of the publicly funded health services. In the main these include general practitioner (GP) based services, hospital based services, community health services, and mental health services.

The term primary care is sometimes used to refer to GP practice based care, though strictly speaking the breadth of primary care is wider and also includes other commonly experienced mainstream services with ready access in the community, including community pharmacy, optometry, and dental practice services. The scope of community health services is less tightly defined administratively, but usually refers to the 'therapies', community nursing specialties, and other services in the community; for example, physiotherapy, occupational therapy, speech and language therapy, community nursing, health visiting, school nursing, dietetics, podiatry, and other health services as might be appropriate in the community.

Hospital-based provision generally relates to inpatient care, outpatient care, and more specialist investigations and support. This is also the setting of accident and emergency departments, which are often seen as the emergency front door of hospitals with such a department. Ambulance services are also closely aligned to this very visible part of local health services. Mental health services involve a range of services provided from several settings, including GP practice based care, community-based mental health services, hospital-based care, and more specialist secure settings as needed. Mental health services provision is a clear example of how components of care for a cohort of people can involve a range of services spanning several service settings (not unlike many pathways of care for those with other chronic conditions or multi-morbidity). In addition, patients may also need to access other services outside of health services, e.g. from social care and the voluntary sector.

It is worth noting at this point that social care is currently funded on a different basis to health services, although patient care journeys may require input from both. Although some aspects of social care are publicly funded on a population basis (via local authority budgets), there are elements that are means tested and self-funded.

Terminology: Primary, secondary, and tertiary care

These terms are sometimes used with reference to healthcare in administrative discussions. They are described here to help with fluency when needed, however in situations where their use risks more confusion than clarity, it may be easier to just be specific about which services we are referring to (e.g. a diabetes clinic or a genitourinary clinic). Access to different types of health services has traditionally been described within a hierarchy of primary, secondary, and tertiary care. This generally reflects how the population accesses the services and to an extent, how specialized the services are.

A key feature of primary care services is that they are a first port of call. In the English health system this refers to the level of care that is directly accessible by patients. GP practice services are the example that comes to most people's minds. The expertise deployed at this level needs to be more generalist in nature but there is no less expertise that is required in order to sort out the important from the less important and the urgent from the less urgent issues that need healthcare attention. There is an element of a gatekeeper role, in that primary care will try to deal with the conditions and situations that can be managed safely at this level, and can refer patients on to other parts of the system for further assistance as necessary. It tends to deal with individual needs earlier on in the development of a condition and has an ongoing role to play in the patient's overall health. In England, several services come under the description of primary care services for oversight by NHS England, namely GP services, community pharmacy services, dentistry, and optometry (optician services).[3]

A feature of secondary care services is that other than emergency care, a referral from primary care is usually needed to access secondary care services. The referral is usually from a GP, though not always so. Services at secondary care level are specialized, in the sense that the expertise deployed draws from a more focused spectrum than that of primary care. Examples of secondary care services are orthopaedics, paediatrics, ophthalmology, neurology, general surgery, general medicine, and many others. Traditionally the term secondary care has been used to refer to the care received as an inpatient or in the outpatients setting of a hospital. However, this can be an incomplete description, as although many of these services are hospital based, many secondary care services are also delivered from non-hospital premises in community settings, for example community paediatrics and mental health services.

Some hospital sites will also be providers of some tertiary care services. Tertiary care describes increasingly specialist care, for example hyperacute stroke care and cardiac surgery. Not all hospital sites will provide tertiary care, and these services might only be available on a larger conurbation footprint. Some of these tertiary care level services will also be deemed 'specialized services', a list of services which are coordinated at a national level (with regional teams), and there is a nationally prescribed list of these.[4]

The group of services commonly understood or referred to as community health services also need to be considered. Although sometimes grouped alongside primary care, they actually provide a supportive layer of care to all the main primary, secondary, and tertiary care descriptions, and can also serve a diagnostic purpose in their own right (e.g. through physiotherapy and speech therapy consultations).

Informal self-care and lay care by family and friends also lie outside of these descriptions, though both are central and adjunctive to overall care experienced by the population.

The 'behind-the-scenes' components

Behind-the-scenes of the more visible elements of a health system, work is needed to make sure that the funds available are used to secure a range of services for the population. This is the work of commissioning. As a generic description, commissioning organizations or 'commissioners' are the fund-holding layer for the population. Essentially, they hold the funds on behalf of a population and are responsible for acquiring a comprehensive range of services for its citizens.

The work of commissioning encompasses a range of activities including planning, prioritizing, assessing outcomes of care, and general decision-making to ensure funds translate into services to address the health needs of the population. It is a mechanism through which available resources are translated to health services for population health gain.

Commissioning is more than the transactional task of paying for services which the term purchasing might imply. Given the whole population context, a working definition of commissioning is, 'a set of purposeful activities to secure quality services for a population to improve health outcomes and reduce health inequalities within finite resources'. There is more about these activities in Chapter 4.

There are particular features of health services and healthcare need which further explain why this intermediary layer of work is needed in some shape or form in a publicly funded system with population-wide coverage. Firstly, there is information asymmetry in healthcare; that is, knowledge about healthcare is not equally held between the users of healthcare and the providers of healthcare. It would be unreasonable to expect all citizens to have in-depth knowledge of the full range of health services they would need to buy or be covered for as part of a comprehensive range of services for themselves or their family's potential needs. Because of this asymmetry, some type of intermediary layer acting on behalf of citizens will be needed to secure a range of services for the population as a whole. Secondly the need for healthcare can be unpredictable for individuals. Although the chance of requiring a costly specific health intervention may be low, the cost impact of this for an individual, if this happened, may be severe. In those circumstances, some collective risk pooling arrangement is sensible. An intermediary layer has the capacity to smooth out such unpredictable risks at a population level. Thirdly, in a publicly funded system, the resources for taking care of the population's health are finite, and if access to healthcare is to be sensitive to needs (as opposed to metering out the same aliquot of care to all individuals regardless of individual need) some kind of intermediary layer is required to facilitate the effectiveness and efficiency of doing this.

Commissioning structures usually comprise a local commissioning layer of coordination and one or more regional or sub-regional tiers before a central national tier (Department of Health or equivalent), from which health service funds originate. These structures between central government and local commissioners may have some commissioning functions of their own, but generally (implicitly or explicitly), they serve to oversee governance of local systems. Duties of such regional or sub-regional tiers can vary in emphasis, and different roles have been prominent at different points in time (including for example strategic leadership, performance management, administrative oversight, roles as a commissioner of services, workforce development, or hybrids of these).

Origins and iterations of commissioning of health services in England

This behind-the-scenes function is not new. The need for health service funds from central government to go through an intermediary layer (or layers) on its way to the frontline of delivery in health services is longstanding. In theory the intermediate layer is where more locally focused decisions can be made about the distribution of central funds to the various local providers. From 1974 to 1990, the emphasis of this layer by modern standards would have been to directly administer the hospital system, secure services with local primary care providers, and generally to administer a local system. Hospitals were directly managed units and GP practices were independent contractors, albeit to the NHS (through the Family Practitioner Committees, which later became the Family Health Services Authorities). Community health and ambulance services which had been administered by the local authorities previously also came under the NHS umbrella in 1974.

In 1989, the government white paper, 'Working for Patients', introduced the 'purchaser-provider' split, delineating differences in responsibilities between the funders (purchasers) and the deliverers of care (providers).[5] This introduced the 'internal market', a so-called market within the NHS system. District health authorities came into being, as did 'GP fundholding' (GP practices could apply for a budget to purchase hospital services for their patients), and hospitals could apply to be NHS trusts in this internal market model.[6] Thus 1990 saw the beginning of the development of more formal distinctions between the purchaser and provider aspects of health services. The district health authorities and family health services authorities later merged to form health authorities, with a combined role for securing hospital, community health, and primary care services. By the end of that decade, devolution in the UK meant that the respective UK nations' health systems diverged. By 2002, in England, the local commissioners, the health authorities, and their fundholding GP subsidiary arrangements had been abolished, and eventually primary care trusts (PCTs) and the strategic health authorities (SHAs), which the PCTs reported to, became the intermediate layer.[7] Involvement of clinical input into this layer would be through professional executive committees (PECs) which were subcommittees aligned to each PCT. By the closing years of the decade, the development of commissioning in health services was underlined by the World Class Commissioning (WCC) initiative in the English NHS.[8] The latter aimed to support and assess the development of health services commissioning work of the PCTs at the time. A couple of annual cycles of this were completed across the English PCT system. In 2010 the then coalition government announced a reorganization of almost all aspects of the behind-the-scenes NHS infrastructure. This was later to become the Health and Social Care Act 2012.[9] As part of this, the WCC initiative was discontinued as PCTs and SHAs were abolished and eventually (with some interim naming conventions), the new Clinical Commissioning Groups (CCGs) emerged as the main new local health service commissioners, along with NHS England, to whom the former would also report. Local public health department functions which had been part of PCTs were to move into local government administrations, and along with that some local health services would also be commissioned from there. Together these new local commissioners (CCGs, NHS England, and local authority public health departments) would pick up the commissioning of health services that the previous PCTs had undertaken.

The Health and Social Care Act 2012 had thrown up a greater array of local commissioning arrangements for different components of health pathways than had previously been the case. A patient pathway involving several health service components for different aspects of care could now involve services commissioned by a number of different commissioners. For example maternity and children's services would now involve the commissioning input of CCGs (for maternity care, neonatal care, paediatrics, and later also for GP practice care), NHS England (for antenatal screening programmes, childhood immunizations, specialized children's services), and local authority public health departments (for school nursing, childhood measurement programme, and later, health visiting). This greater complexity increased the risk of fragmented responses to pathway issues experienced by patients. Towards 2018, there was increasing focus on improving connections between different components of patient care, which led to more explicit development of integrated models of care.[10] Notably, this did not necessarily come with any changes in accountability arrangements of the individual commissioners. Only time will tell whether that too is needed to strengthen integrated approaches.

Who commissions what?

In essence, there is a range of services providing care in different settings and a number of organizations holding funds, the latter being the commissioners through which the money passes to reach frontline organizations. The details of who commissions what will depend on the arrangements of the day. What can be gleaned is that the intermediary layer takes on the role of securing services for the local population, and has done so with varying degrees of explicitness about specifications and contracting over time in the English system. That said, the aim of securing health gain for the population through these efforts remains pertinent whatever the structures of the day.

For illustration, Table 2.1 shows arrangements introduced after the Health and Social Care Act 2012 and arrangements from earlier periods for interest. It illustrates how the span of services to be secured has remained constant although the commissioning (fundholding) arrangements can change over time.

After the 2012 Act came into force, the bulk of health services commissioning for local populations was via the CCGs, as the latter became responsible for commissioning the majority of hospital, mental health, community health services, and aspects of GP practice care. In effect, they would commission all NHS funded services not prescribed for NHS England to commission. Interestingly the NHS England tier that CCGs reported to, would also themselves commission a discrete range of health services. These were usually services where a common contract could be applied to a larger footprint, for example primary care services, cancer screening programmes, and nationally defined specialized services. In addition, some local health services would also be commissioned by local authorities. These latter services would be funded through a public health grant from central government.[11] Examples included sexual health, smoking cessation, 'NHS Health Checks', school nursing services, and others as this evolved.

Subsequently therefore, central funds for health services (from the Department of Health or equivalent) would flow down various routes via commissioners to reach providers. Suffice to say, whatever the behind-the-scenes commissioning arrangements of the day, it is important to remember that the services for the end-users (patients, carers, and citizens) needs to be thought of as a coherent pathway; when working in any aspect of such a system, one needs to be aware of this bigger picture.

Table 2.1 Health service commissioning organizations in England and service commissioning responsibilities (1990–2018)

Commissioning organization		Service type						
		General practice services	Other primary care: dentistry, optometry, pharmacy	Hospital-based services	Community health services	Local mental health services	Specialized services	Screening and immunization
District Health Authority*	1990–2002[6]	✓	✓	✓	✓	✓	✓	✓
Primary Care Trust (PCT)**	2002–2012[7]	✓	✓	✓	✓	✓	✓	✓
Clinical Commissioning Group (CCG)	At April 2013[3,9]	✓		✓	✓	✓		
NHS England	2013–	✓	✓	✓	✓	✓	✓	
Local authority public health departments		✓	✓		✓			✓

* Accountable via Regional Offices to the Department of Health. Within this era there were also subsidiary GP fundholding arrangements whereby GP practices had responsibility for some aspects of their practice population spending (e.g. outpatient referrals). Some variants of this covered multiple practice populations and a wider range of responsibilities, but ultimately the accountability for securing services for the population rested with the district health authority layer.

** Accountable via Strategic Health Authorities to the Department of Health.

N.B. The table is illustrative, local arrangements may vary since 2013.

Constancy of the population approach

From the longer term viewpoint, there has been longstanding balancing and rebalancing of 'top-down' (more centralized, larger footprint strategy) and 'bottom-up' (more localized, smaller population footprint commissioning) approaches over time in the publicly funded English health system. This reflects varying attempts to balance sufficient local view, engagement, and innovation, with retaining sufficient centralized control for overview, economies of scale, and to provide an accountable governance layer for decisions affecting larger footprints. Whether future blends of locally evolved and 'top-down' centrally directed structures will achieve that optimum equilibrium remains to be seen.

And so commissioning continues to take place in this constantly evolving context. Structural names may change, but the underlying endeavour remains the same, to secure quality services for a population in an equitable way that improves health within finite resources. Workable care pathways that make practical sense to patients and their carers so that they can use them effectively will always be needed. People will still have needs for effective services to manage a range of conditions. The basic principles of using a population approach to securing services are likely to be pertinent long into the future.

Whatever the local commissioning structures of the day, as long as there is a population basis to secure services for, the principles of a population approach to health services decision-making will be pertinent. Further, the underpinning concepts of a population approach remain, even if currently existing roles of commissioners and providers become more closely aligned, as long as the purpose remains to secure services on a population basis.

Reflection

On a practical level, with these visible and behind-the-scenes structures in mind, how familiar are you with your local arrangements?

References

1. Ham C. *Health Policy in Britain*. Third Edition. MacMillan Press Limited, 1992.
2. Department of Health. Public health in local government: Commissioning responsibilities. Gateway reference 16747. December 2011.

3. NHS Commissioning Board. Commissioning fact sheet for clinical commissioning groups. July 2012. Available at: https://www.england.nhs.uk/wp-content/uploads/2012/07/fs-ccg-respon.pdf

4. NHS England. Manual for Prescribed Specialised Services 2018/19. September 2018. Available at: https://www.england.nhs.uk/wp-content/uploads/2017/10/prescribed-specialised-services-manual.pdf

5. Department for Health and Social Security, HMSO. Working for Patients. 1989.

6. HMSO. National Health Service and Community Care Act 1990.

7. Department of Health. Shifting the balance of power within the NHS, securing delivery. July 2001.

8. Department of Health. World class commissioning assurance handbook, year 2. Gateway reference 12458. September 2009.

9. HMSO. Health and Social Care Act 2012.

10. NHS. The NHS Long Term Plan. January 2019. Available at: https://www.longtermplan.nhs.uk/publication/nhs-long-term-plan/

11. Department of Health. The new public health role of local authorities. Gateway reference 17876. 2012.

3

Commissioning Needs a Population Perspective

The point of a health service is to make a positive difference to the population's health. To do this the resources available need to reach those who need it, in a needs-led and equitable manner. The 'commissioning machinery' in a health system that secures these services must therefore take a population health gain approach as part of its strategic and day-to-day considerations. This chapter will describe how the commissioning of health services is enabled and enhanced when there is active use of the population perspective as part of the process.

This requires a 'big picture' vision of health and health services, as well as working knowledge of what commissioning entails. You will already have a feel for the latter from Chapter 2, so this chapter will focus on the population perspective as relevant to commissioning. Considering the wide range of health issues a commissioner may come across, it is unlikely that anyone would have all the information they need, all the time, already in their heads. Compiling useful orientation on a topic will usually involve some enquiries and effort. The key is to have some bearings to help guide you through the population-wide considerations that will inevitably come your way as a commissioner. This chapter aims to help you get up and running on this. It introduces a basic format to open up any health topic to a population approach. The perspectives can be applied to many guises of health service discussions.

Main points to be familiar with . . .

- Key perspectives for scoping the 'big picture' using a population approach to healthcare problem-solving.
- The area of commonality between 'big picture' health practice (public health practice) and commissioning practice is essential in commissioning for health gain.

Commissioning and a Population Approach to Health Services Decision-Making. Julie Sin, Oxford University Press (2020). © Oxford University Press. DOI: 10.1093/oso/9780198840732.001.0001

Interdependency of 'big picture' health and commissioning skills

First we need to appreciate the essential relationship between the population health gain approach and commissioning efforts. This is illustrated in Figure 3.1.

The shaded area in Figure 3.1 indicates where a population perspective is applied to the processes of health services commissioning. In this overlap, evidence-based knowledge of health and healthcare, and contextual knowledge of healthcare systems, is applied to considerations and decision-making for a population. This is relevant to many aspects of commissioning and steers efforts towards health gain. Health gain refers to increases in the health of a population as a result of effective actions (for example less illness, less premature deaths, or other measurable improvement).

Not only does using a population perspective facilitate a needs-led approach to planning and decision-making, it also allows a fuller breadth of opportunities for protecting and improving health to be recognized, from upstream actions and treatments to end-of-life care. Such a 'big picture' approach also allows insight into the consequences for other parts of the system (positive or negative) to be recognized when resources are used in one part of the system rather than another.

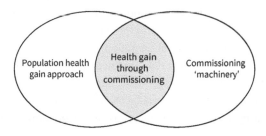

With its inherent big picture health skills:
• Evidence-based approach to disease prevention, treatment and care in the population.
• Relevance to planning, prioritization and evaluation of health services.
• Helps to steer commissioning decisions towards health gain.

With its commissioning skills:
• The business processes and skills needed for securing quality services for the population.
• Including needs-led planning, prioritization, procurement, contracting, and evaluation.

Figure 3.1 Interdependency of big picture health skills and commissioning skills

In practice this means adopting some key vantage points when trying to solve health system problems.

Key facets of a population approach to healthcare

The following facets can be used to compile context and discern the opportunities for effective action for a population. Each is a different vantage point to understand the topic in-hand from a population perspective. They comprise:

a. Epidemiological context and the natural history of the condition.
b. Effective preventive opportunities.
c. Reduction of inequalities in access to, and outcomes of, services.
d. Whole system, care pathway considerations.

You could think of the acronym 'EPICS' to help you remember these, namely: Epidemiological story, Preventive opportunities, Inequalities reduction, and the Care pathway and System considerations. The format can be used to scope a health issue quickly. An evidence-based approach is used throughout.

Depending on the information you already have, you might want to apply one or two of these vantage points, or consider them all. Essentially, by exploring these perspectives for commissioning, it will help answer important commissioning questions such as, 'what is this condition and why is it a problem?', 'what is the natural course of the condition and the earliest effective points to make a difference?', 'what do we know about causation?', 'what are the effective things that could work in my area?', 'what data do I need to understand the picture?', and 'how to contribute effectively to reducing health inequalities?'.

Even using just one or two of these facets to scope an issue will enhance your commissioning work. You can always go back to do more as time allows.

Natural history of the condition and epidemiological context

In essence this is the big picture of a health matter. The natural history of a condition provides orientation about its natural course over time (for example whether it is a self-limiting condition, acute or chronic, benign or severe, or a combination of these); whether it is a major cause of early deaths, illness, or disability; and the longer term outlook for people affected. In the clinical setting, knowing the natural history of a condition helps with considering diagnosis, treatment options, and preventive opportunities for the individual patient. For the commissioner of health services, gathering an overall understanding of this (not necessarily at the level of detail needed for making a diagnosis and coordinating individual treatment) helps to understand whether it is an important condition, and if necessary, to begin considering the effective actions at a population level. Epidemiology contributes understanding about the distribution and determinants of health problems. Distribution refers to the timing, place, and groups of people affected, and what can be learnt from those. Determinants refer to the factors that influence health. Thus epidemiological context adds to the commissioning picture by framing the health issue in population terms, for example to gauge the number of people affected, if there are any particular patterns in their distribution, and what may be the main known determinants. Together, the natural history of the condition and the epidemiological context help to assess whether this is an important health issue (and if so, why important), and its impact on the population. This facet thus helps with setting the scene for your work and complements any local contextual knowledge which may have triggered the issue.

To incorporate this facet in your work, typically you might summarize what you can of the following:

- Why is this an important condition (or group of conditions) in the population? For example, is it a significant cause of illness, disability, or premature mortality?
- How common is it? For example, what is the incidence (new cases per 100,000 per year) or prevalence (cases per 100,000 population at a point in time)? And so, how many people does this affect in our population? How many of those are we aware of?
- What are the main known risk factors?
- What is known about the natural course of the condition?
- How does our population compare with others? For example, similar demographic populations, or the country as a whole.
- Are any population subgroups at higher risk than others?

Preventive opportunities

Taking this vantage point helps to consider the opportunities across the course of a condition's development to reduce the burden of ill health now and/or in the future. It involves the consideration of a range of effective preventive opportunities, from pre-illness, early detection to alter the course of the condition, to effective treatment options and ongoing care as relevant. Be aware that although not all conditions can be prevented from occurring they may still be amenable to opportunities to prevent further deterioration or recurrence (hence effective treatment opportunities are included within this consideration). Whether such preventive opportunities are easy to identify or not will depend on the issue in hand. A holistic approach is advised to help identify these (more on this in Chapter 7). Attention to this facet will help you to consider a range of opportunities to deal with the condition of interest when allocating resources to a care pathway.

To make use of this facet, summarize what you can of the potentially effective intervention points with respect to your topic of interest. It will give you a picture of the range of opportunities or act as a guide of areas to explore.

Inequalities in access and outcomes

This is the third, but no less important, 'stop and think' point in the basic orientation to a population approach to health services. Attention to this facet helps to ensure that commissioning has regard to equity as it improves services. The concept of equity in this context refers to equal opportunities for equal health needs.

Across a population, some variations in access to health services would be expected, even with equitable access to care. For example, we know that on average, people over 65 years of age receive more care from stroke services than people from younger age groups, as stroke is largely a degenerative condition for which risk increases with age. This picture would therefore not be unexpected. However, if there were variations in the access to, or outcomes from health services that were not related to health need and where amenable action were possible, these would be unwarranted variations in access and outcomes. For example, if there were variations by geography or by levels of deprivation in the access to cancer services, these would be a concern.

Reducing inequities in health is of course a big topic in its own right and is explored with respect to commissioning in a later chapter (Chapter 14). For now, as a key facet of a population approach to commissioning, it is suffice to say that commissioners should be aware that aiming to reduce inequities in access and outcomes of care is a legitimate concern for population healthcare effectiveness, and that as a commissioner one should consider this in planning as well as in the appraisal of any health service issues we may come across.

When dealing with any unwarranted variation in access or outcomes in the population, the aim is of course to 'level up', that is to improve the experience of the worse off to help reduce the gap, not to diminish the experience of anyone else.

To incorporate this vantage point in your work, typically you might summarize what you can of any routine monitoring or other practical measures you have in place to assess or mitigate against unwarranted inequalities in access and outcomes for the service you are considering. Or indeed, identify where these steps need to be in place.

Whole care pathway and system considerations

This last facet helps to consider the bigger picture of the health and care services in the system that is relevant to the individuals with the condition of interest. A whole care pathway approach can be used to consider the contributions of the various upstream components, primary care, self-care, community, and hospital setting components relevant to any condition pathway. This organizational context is complementary to all the epidemiological and effectiveness information you have gathered so far.

You can use this organizational settings perspective to capture any further opportunities to improve health not already identified using the other perspectives, or indeed to help identify any gaps in these assets locally. It is a useful additional perspective for scoping health and care system issues that cannot be easily disentangled using a single health condition pathway (for example 'children's health services', where a vast array of conditions and issues may be included, or 'winter pressures' on health services, which is a system issue rather than a single condition).

The care pathway or care journey perspective also underpins an important point about pathways. That is, it is the *overall effectiveness* of the pathway that matters for population outcomes. For example, you may have the most effective and efficacious medicines in the world to improve outcomes from a classic ischaemic stroke (a stroke due to blockage of a blood vessel supplying the brain tissue) but if the patients who can benefit from this cannot reach the hospital on time to be assessed and given treatment, then the outcomes of the pathway as a whole will not be as effective as expected. Using a whole care pathway approach helps to understand the practical issues at hand, and identify options for improvement in the service response to the condition you are considering.

To make use of this facet in your scoping, typically you might summarize what you can of any important interdependencies that your topic of interest has with other services. For example, the interdependency of maternity with neonatal services, general surgery with anaesthetics, or the care of frail elderly patients with many community services. In many modern health service arrangements, there may be a number of different commissioners involved in securing different parts of the pathway, so it is important to have awareness of the 'patient's journey' with their condition, and who the different commissioning organizations (commissioners) involved in this care pathway are in your area.

Evidence-based approach at the population level

The use of an evidence-based approach should underpin the use of the above facets in your scoping. Basic familiarity with the purpose of taking an evidence-based approach has been assumed as it is a fundamental part of continuously improving practice. The value of using an evidence-based approach is extensively described in the clinical practice and wider healthcare literature, so it will not be reviewed here per se. The aim of this chapter instead focuses on what one can 'do' with it to help commissioning, rather than its intrinsic value. For convenience however, there follows a definition of the approach, in case needed.

Essentially, an evidence-based approach means making use of the best available evidence to understand the situation, with the aim of improving practice. It is used throughout scientific disciplines, social sciences, and in clinical practice. Whilst it recognizes that there will always be gaps in research evidence for many things and that evidence may not always be black or white in clarity, the approach is an antidote to guard against 'evidence-light' or even 'evidence-free' practice or policy making. In healthcare, the term was initially described with reference to informing decisions about patient care and has since been widely accepted as being an informative contribution to many different levels of decision-making. At the population level, where most healthcare planning and buying of services is considered, an evidence-based approach is just as applicable as it is at the clinical practice level.

The original description of evidence-based practice from Sackett et al[1] as, 'the conscientious, explicit and judicious use of current best evidence to make decisions about the care of individual patients', remains the basis of commonly used definitions of the evidence-based approach in clinical practice. The following working definition is offered as an approach which can be applied at the population level. It is adapted from Sackett's description of evidence-based practice in the clinical setting, for population level practice.

Evidence-based approach for population level practice: The conscientious and explicit use of evidence in informing and making decisions about the care of the population and its individuals. It means integrating expertise about the local population context with the best available external evidence from systematic research.

Thus, an evidence-based approach is as relevant on a population level as it is at the clinical level of decision-making. Note the mention of local population context; that contextual knowledge about the environment we are working in is complementary to knowledge from the research evidence and numerical statistics. It includes wider understanding about the population and its local health system in which decisions are taken. Gathering such contextual knowledge may seem a messy and rather unscientific endeavour compared to carefully prepared journal publications and hard quantitative data, but it is this context that may make the difference between a meaningful discussion that leads to effective action and one that does not. For decision-making, context is essential. A structured approach to gathering the context and evidence in one place can facilitate the work of using it all to make a difference for health.

Scoping a topic

You can use the key facets described as a basic structure to scope any health or healthcare related topic. The level of detail you want to achieve is up to you and could range from making some preliminary prompts to a full-blown summary. Boxes 3.1 and 3.2 are examples.

Box 3.1 **Example of scoping a topic—Bowel Cancer**

Imagine you are part of a fact-finding group considering how to re-duce bowel cancer deaths in your area. Your group serves a popu-lation in the north of the country where cancer incidence in general is higher than the national average. The group consider the points below to help understand what more can be done with respect to bowel cancer, who does what, and which organizations need to work together. The group is multidisciplinary, and everyone knows something but no one will know everything. It has access to all avail-able web-based resources as well as the knowledge they bring with them. They use best practice guidance, systematic reviews, and rou-tinely available statistics to guide them. After an initial meeting and a short email exchange afterwards, they have gathered the following orientation.

Epidemiology and natural history of the condition

Bowel cancer (colorectal cancer) remains one of the three most common causes of cancer deaths for males and females in England. Early detection and treatment improves survival rates.

The commonest type is adenocarcinoma of the bowel (>95%) arising from gland cells in the bowel wall.[2]

Symptoms can include a change in bowel habit, pain, bleeding, un-explained weight loss, or there may be few symptoms depending on its location in the bowel. Around half of people diagnosed with colorectal cancer survive for five years or more after diagnosis.

Over three-quarters of cases occur in the over-65 age group and are more common in males than females. Incidence rates of colorectal cancers (rates of new cancers) in England was 84.4 and 55.4 cases per 100,000 for males and females respectively in 2016 (age-standardized). There has been a slight decrease in deaths from bowel cancer over the 2005 to 2016 period. The introduction of the national screening pro-gramme for colorectal cancer may have contributed to the latter.[3]

The main known risk factors are increasing age, dietary and life-style factors (diet higher in processed and red meat and lower in fibre, alcohol, smoking, and obesity), family history of bowel cancer, and in-flammatory bowel disease.[2]

Preventive opportunities
Reduction of dietary and lifestyle risk factors in the population

Opportunities to increase fibre in the diet (cereal fibre and whole grains in particular)[4], moderating consumption of processed and red meat and impact of alcohol consumption. Benefits of physical activity, maintaining a healthy weight, and smoking cessation.[2]

Earlier detection of the disease when it is more amenable to treatment

In England the National Screening Committee weighs up the benefit and harms of population screening programmes before a screening programme is rolled out on a population basis to screen asymptomatic individuals of average risk. In England the NHS bowel cancer screening programme offers a non-invasive screening test two yearly for eligible age groups (using a faecal occult blood (FOB) test or increasingly the faecal immunochemical test (FIT) test on a stool sample). A positive test result leads to an invitation for colonoscopy examination of the large bowel for confirmation of disease or otherwise. An additional one-off flexible sigmoidoscopy test to examine the lower portion of the large bowel is being introduced across England.[5,6]

Another earlier detection opportunity involves the screening and review of higher risk groups (people with Crohn's disease, ulcerative colitis, or relevant family history).[7]

Effective treatment services and ongoing care

Prompt diagnosis and access to appropriate care, whether cancer has been detected through a screening programme or has presented through other routes.[8] Care related to living with bowel cancer, and palliative care to lessen any day-to-day disability.

Reducing inequalities in access and outcomes

Raising awareness about diet and lifestyle opportunities to prevent bowel and other cancers, and about early presentation if there are symptoms of concern, should be population-wide, and additionally targeted if there is a locality or cohort of concern.

As all eligible people in the population are invited for screening using a systematic call-recall system, this reduces the risk of inequities in access to screening. Consider what further routine statistics are available to help assess local access and outcomes of care and whether they could be more equitable (for example with respect to access to screening, access to treatment, and emergency admissions for cancer).

Other care pathway and system considerations

Organizations that are responsible for securing the provision of the different aspects of the pathway are: commissioners of primary care, screening programmes (including laboratory components), gastro-enterology, surgical specialties, pathology, oncology, radiology, palliative care, national and local health improvement components.

Not only have the group gathered the above, they can begin to see aspects that they did not have line of sight of on a day-to-day basis. They are now in a better position to interpret and assess issues in the system or any isolated pieces of data in context. This makes for more collaborative discussions and problem-solving. Having scoped, they decide to see what further information is available about how the local pathway is working. For example local screening uptake, premature mortality (deaths in <75 year olds), percentage of cancers presenting at an early stage compared to national average or relevant peer populations.

Box 3.2 **Example of scoping a topic—Stroke Care**

Imagine for example that you are part of a multidisciplinary group involved in reviewing and designing stroke services for your local population of 250,000 people. You have come together to consider how to reduce incidence of strokes and the resulting disability in your area. The group decide to pool their understanding and consider the elements below to help understand what can be done and who does what.

Epidemiology and natural history of the condition

Strokes are a major cause of premature mortality in the UK.[9] They can occur at any age, but increasing age is an important risk factor, with about three-quarters of strokes occurring in people aged

65 years and over. A stroke or a cerebrovascular accident (CVA) occurs when blood flow to the brain is interrupted. Strokes can be ischaemic (85% of strokes) or haemorrhagic (15%).[10] Ischaemic strokes arise when a blood vessel supplying the brain becomes blocked. This may have become blocked suddenly due to a clot arising within fatty deposits in the blood vessel, or from a clot (embolus) that has travelled from elsewhere in the circulation. Clot-dissolving treatment (thrombolysis) given early in these strokes can improve outcomes. Haemorrhagic strokes are less common and result from a bleed on the surface of the brain. Outcomes from haemorrhagic strokes are poorer. Overall, one in eight strokes are fatal within 30 days of the event.[11]

Incidence rates of first stroke were 1.13 per 1,000 in England in 2016 (age-standardized to European population), and strokes were slightly more common in males than females (1.20 compared to 1.00 per 1,000). Incidence decreased a little over the ten years 2007 to 2016. However the mean age at first stroke has reduced from an average of 72.4 to 70.6 years in the ten years to 2016.[12]

The main known modifiable risk factors are hypertension, diabetes, atrial fibrillation, tobacco smoking, alcohol consumption, sedentary lifestyle, apolipoprotein (cholesterol) ratios, and abdominal obesity.[13]

Preventive opportunities
Before event
Awareness raising and advice about reducing modifiable behavioural and metabolic risk factors through lifestyle should be population-wide. Opportunities to improve high blood pressure detection and management, atrial fibrillation detection and management, diabetes control, reducing smoking prevalence in the population, walking and physical activity.

In addition, there may be specific cardiovascular risk factor checks such as the NHS Health Checks programme for asymptomatic 40–74 year olds, though ongoing evaluation is needed to optimize these opportunities.[17]

For people already known to have a higher risk of stroke (e.g. patients with known cardiovascular disease, diabetes, sickle cell disease, and other predisposing conditions), action at an individual level to reduce modifiable risk factors.

During acute event

Prompt diagnosis of stroke, stroke unit care, and appropriate timely use of thrombolysis treatment reduces mortality and residual disability compared with conservative treatment. Stroke care should cover the breadth of hyper-acute care, acute care, and rehabilitation.[10,14,15]

After event

Rehabilitation to optimize physical and cognitive function. Medications to reduce recurrence of CVA.[10,16]

Reducing inequalities in access and outcomes

Awareness raising of modifiable risk factors and effective stroke diagnosis and care should be accessible to all in the population. If cardiovascular health checks are available to asymptomatic population, (e.g. 'NHS Health Checks'), an approach that reaches all sections of the population increases the effectiveness of the programme and this will need ongoing monitoring.[17] Consider what further routine statistics are available to help assess local access and outcomes of care and whether they could be more equitable.

Other care pathway and system considerations

Organizations that are responsible for securing different aspects of a comprehensive pathway include: commissioners of primary care, acute stroke services and rehabilitation, social care, ambulance services, national and local awareness raising, and other opportunities in the pre-illness phase to offer blood pressure, diabetes, and atrial fibrillation identification and management as part of a local pathway.

The extent of the opportunities is now clearer. Having scoped, the group decide to gather more information about how the local pathways are working to inform their commissioning. For example, they look at the take-up rate of health checks, the detection and management of high blood pressure across GP practices, and find ways to make feasible improvements. They will also look at national audit data of their local stroke unit.

Naming convention for the 'big picture' health and commissioning overlap

The area of overlap in Figure 3.1 represents the opportunities for commissioning with a population approach in the healthcare system. The common goal here is to make sure health services lead to health gains for the population. This area of commonality is an integral part of both commissioning and of public health practice.

Achieving health gain from the healthcare system is a core part of public health practice, and this area of work is known as 'Healthcare Public Health' (HCPH) within the public health specialty. It is concerned with health service effectiveness at the population level and the quality of services. From a commissioning perspective, the equivalent could be thought of as 'commissioning for health gain', that is when a whole population perspective is actively used as an integral part of commissioning.

This interconnecting area of practice provides essential context for decision-making at a population level. As a branch of applied medicine, it may be easier for some clinicians to think of the healthcare public health practice as 'health systems medicine'. Colleagues with an organizational management leaning may see the work in this arena as 'big picture healthcare management', or 'population healthcare management'. Work in this arena is indeed multidisciplinary, and familiarity with big picture health concepts ('public health' concepts) and the mechanics of commissioning helps. It needs to be acknowledged, but probably does not matter, that different originating methodologies might refer to this intersecting area of work as slightly different things (there are examples from other spheres of work where naming conventions for areas of commonality may differ slightly due to different methodological origins, such as in the fields of architecture and civil engineering, or art and design). The important thing is that the strategic importance of this area of commonality is recognized and valued, and unnecessary barriers are not put in the way for overlapping disciplines to work together for better health and care in the population.

Reflection

If you were to use the 'EPICS' approach in a discussion or decision you have been involved with recently, how different would your starting point be? Would it have changed any of your contributions to the discussion?

References

1. Sackett DL, Rosenberg WM, Gray JA, Haynes RB, Richardson WS. Evidence based medicine: what it is and what it isn't. *BMJ* 1996;312:71.
2. Thrumurthy SG, Thrumurthy SS, Gilbert CE, Ross P, Haji A. Colorectal adenocarcinoma: risks, prevention and diagnosis. *BMJ* 2016;354:i3590.
3. Office for National Statistics. Cancer registration statistics, England: 2016. Statistical Bulletin. June 2018. Available at: https://www.ons.gov.uk/peoplepopulationandcommunity/healthandsocialcare/conditionsanddiseases/bulletins/cancerregistrationstatisticsengland/final2016
4. Aune D, Chan DS, Lau R. Dietary fibre, whole grains and risk of colorectal cancer: systematic review and dose-response meta-analysis of prospective studies. *BMJ* 2011;343:d6617.
5. NHS England. Bowel Cancer Screening. Updated February 2018. Available at: https://www.nhs.uk/conditions/bowel-cancer-screening
6. NHS England. Bowel cancer screening: programme overview. Updated November 2018. Available at: https://www.gov.uk/guidance/bowel-cancer-screening-programme-overview
7. NICE. Colorectal cancer prevention: colonoscopic surveillance in adults with ulcerative colitis, Crohn's disease or adenomas. Clinical Guideline [CG118]. March 2011. Available at: https://www.nice.org.uk/guidance/cg118
8. NICE. Colorectal cancer: diagnosis and management. Clinical Guideline[CG131]. Updated December 2014. Available at: https://www.nice.org.uk/guidance/cg131
9. Steel N, Ford JA, Newton JN, Davis ACJ, Vos T, Naghavi M et al. Changes in health in the countries of the UK and 150 English Local Authority areas 1990–2016: a systematic analysis for the Global Burden of Disease Study 2016. *Lancet* 2018;392:1647–1661.
10. Royal College of Physicians. National clinical guideline for Stroke Intercollegiate Stroke Working Party, 5th edition. 2016.
11. Bray BD, Cloud GC, James MA et al. Weekly variation in health-care quality by day and time of admission: a nationwide, registry-based, prospective cohort study of acute stroke care. *Lancet*. 2016;388:170–177.
12. PHE publications. Briefing document: first incidence of stroke. Estimates for England 2007 to 2016. Gateway reference 2017613. February 2018.
13. O'Donnell MJ, Chin SL, Rangarajan S et al. Global and regional effects of potentially modifiable risk factors associated with acute stroke in 32 countries (INTERSTROKE): a case-control study. *Lancet* 2016; 388:761–775.
14. NICE. Stroke in adults. Quality standard (QS2). June 2010, updated April 2016.
15. NICE. Stroke and transient ischaemic attacks in over 16s: diagnosis and initial management. Clinical guideline [CG68]. July 2008, updated March 2017.
16. NICE. Stroke rehabilitation in adults. Clinical Guideline [CG162]. June 2013.
17. Public Health England. Emerging evidence on the NHS health check: findings and recommendations. A report from the Expert Scientific and Clinical Advisory Panel. February 2017.

4
The Basic Commissioning Cycle

This is an orientation for those new to the concept of a commissioning cycle, or a synopsis for those who have experienced parts of the process.

Main points to be familiar with ...

- What is commissioning?
- What are the key parts of a commissioning cycle?
- Commissioning is a multidisciplinary effort.

What is commissioning?

In the health services arena, the term commissioning refers to a collection of processes to secure quality services for the population to help meet its health needs and reduce amenable inequalities in health. This takes place within a context of finite resources available for healthcare and takes into consideration national and local priorities. In practice for an organization, commissioning is a continuous programme of work chunked up into annual cycles ('annual commissioning round') so that proposed spending for the coming year can be checked against resources available. Sometimes the term is used to refer to efforts of securing a specific service for the population, for example, the commissioning of a musculoskeletal service or a sexual health service. Either way the relevance of the main stages and the core purpose of commissioning are the same whether considering a specific service or all the commissioned services of an organization. The different components of commissioning a service are known as a 'Commissioning Cycle'.

Core Purpose of Commissioning To secure quality services for the population, that lead to health gain and reduce health inequalities, within given resources.

Commissioning and a Population Approach to Health Services Decision-Making. Julie Sin, Oxford University Press (2020). © Oxford University Press. DOI: 10.1093/oso/9780198840732.001.0001

What are the key parts of a commissioning cycle?

There are more complicated versions but I have used the following for many years and find it useful for the initiated and uninitiated. In essence the key components of the commissioning cycle boil down to four key stages (see Figure 4.1).

Main stages of the commissioning cycle

In summary these are:

- **Problem definition.** This involves clarifying the pertinent issues and understanding these in the context of existing pathways and the health system as a whole. It involves making use of relevant data, published evidence, and local understanding of the issues. Problem definition identifies the health needs that can be addressed by effective interventions.
- **Prioritization and planning.** Having guiding principles, and workable and consistent decision-making processes to decide priorities is crucial. When a decision to go ahead with a proposed service or intervention has been made, a service specification is needed. This describes what the service needs to deliver to the population and helps interested potential providers to think of ways to meet the requirements.

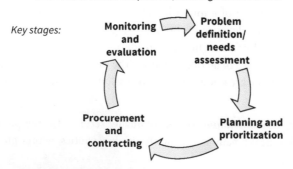

Core purpose:
' To secure quality services for the population that lead to health gain and reduce health inequalities, within given resources.'

Key stages: Monitoring and evaluation → Problem definition/ needs assessment → Planning and prioritization → Procurement and contracting →

Figure 4.1 Commissioning Cycle

- **Procurement and contracting.** Procurement involves understanding the legal and business framework to secure a provider for the service. Contracting is a formal agreement with the chosen provider(s) at agreed cost and quality parameters, including health outcomes.
- **Monitoring and evaluation of outcomes.** This relates to seeking assurance about the continuing quality of the service in place and that it is having the desired impact on health outcomes. It also includes identifying further questions for research.

Learning at any of these stages can feed into the next stage or the next iteration of this process.

Do not worry if it is not always a circular cycle in practice, things can go back and forth a little between some of the earlier stages, but they are the main steps for a structured approach to commissioning. Below are some additional notes to help you make use of the commissioning cycle with confidence.

Problem definition and needs assessment

The essence of this stage is to scope the topic to be tackled and clarify any context about why it is being tackled at this point in time. For example, what has triggered this locally, or is it a national priority, or is there some other reason? This helps to understand the resources you will be able to draw upon and the likelihood of support from the organization and wider system to follow through the commissioning cycle with this topic.

To scope the topic, you may have your own preferred format, if not you can use the 'EPICS' process as a guide from Chapter 3. Your aim here is to orientate the commissioning process to the health issue at hand. You could do this by describing the impact of the condition on people, any effective opportunities to moderate it, and quantifying the local impact if possible. You may have to make reasonable estimates about the latter. You are aiming to identify needs, and effective and cost-effective interventions.

A useful working definition of a *health need* for use in health services commissioning is, 'a health problem for which there is an intervention about which there is strong evidence based on good quality research, that it does more good than harm.'[1] That is, a health need is a problem with an effective solution. This helps to focus on the art of the possible to improve health.

At its most useful, the problem definition stage is the culmination of several perspectives (local context, evidence base for effective interventions, and data to clarify the issues further), rather than viewing the issue as a single piece of data or an expert view, although it all adds to the picture. The practical thing to remember is that the product of this exercise has to enable good decision-making further along the cycle, so it is important to be realistic about the timescales for this work, and that it keeps the commissioning cycle in mind rather than being something done in isolation.

A note for producers of information

Whatever the information available, whether it is nationally or locally produced material, it is likely that much time and effort has been expended in producing this knowledge. To do this justice it needs to translate easily to the commissioning processes if it is to make a difference to health gain through that route. That means that works in isolation of the health service decision-making machinery risk not reaching their full potential of effect if they do not acknowledge the commissioning context. This applies to any local or nationally produced assessments of need, for example, Annual Public Health Reports, Joint Strategic Needs Assessment (JSNA) materials, National Institute for Health and Care Excellence (NICE) materials, and academic papers.

A note for users of information

Build up your familiarity with using an evidence-based approach at a practical level and seek opportunities to nurture this. If it is not part of the induction to your post so far ask for it as part of your ongoing professional and organizational development. Practise using the approach actively and continue to build your experience. You do not need to be an expert when you first get involved with commissioning or service redesign but you do need to be informed about what it is, how to access the various knowledge types, the rudiments of interpreting the quality of the evidence, and how to get more help if needed. If information is not generated in the format you find useful, take the trouble to feed back and be specific about what can be improved.

Prioritization and planning

If there is an effective intervention or service that needs to be in place, you will get to this stage. If it will benefit patients, is effective and cost-effective, an outline business case (or equivalent stage) may be drawn up to summarize the need, the benefits, costs, risks of inaction, and how this fits into the local pathways. This is the beginnings of the planning for implementation.

Be clear about the purpose of any new service to be commissioned or re-designed. Clarity about this goal will help you later. For example, a goal of the service may be for it 'to provide timely access to mental health services for children and adolescents in the population', or 'to provide specialist advice and care for patients with type 1 diabetes, as part of a coherent local pathway'. When it has been agreed, write it down. You will need it later for guiding the service specification and for choosing what measures to monitor.

In reality, not everything that is effective is cost-effective and not all that is cost-effective is affordable. Prioritization is needed to compare all the competing needs for resources and to determine if a proposed course of action can progress past this stage. There may be a formal process of prioritization and decision-making such as an annual commissioning round, or it may be a less structured process performed by delegated officers drawing on a list of guiding principles (the latter may be called an ethical framework for commissioning). Prioritization is discussed further in Chapter 10.

Prioritization may take place *within* a care pathway, that would consider if resources can be released from elsewhere in the pathway to take on a new proposal (e.g. whether feasible to introduce a new testing kit to an existing diabetes pathway). Or prioritization considerations can be *across* many care pathways (e.g. are we investing the 'right' proportions of the total money across the many possible different service pathways such as mental health, cancer, diabetes, and stroke care, etc.). Within-pathway considerations might take place throughout the year so that only the most pertinent developments that cannot be handled that way go through to the annual commissioning process for decisions. But that is not always so and in practice both within- and across-pathway considerations can happen very close together as part of an annual commissioning round.

If a decision is taken to go ahead with commissioning a particular service, a service specification will need to be drawn up. This describes the service you wish to 'buy' or secure for the population. The point of this is to communicate clearly what you want potential 'providers' to deliver for your population. The work you have put into gathering information and context in the previous stages will make your life easier now. In the service specification you will be spelling out the goal of the service, its scope, the population covered, key effective components of the service you need in place, key relationships with other services (for joined up care for the patient), as well as cost parameters. You will also specify the standards expected and describe the monitoring arrangements.

You will have gathered by now that some identified project management input is needed to keep this work on track and this will continue into the next stage of implementation.

Procurement and contracting

Procurement refers to the act of buying or securing goods or services. It includes seeking offers from potential providers to supply goods or do the work and from that, identifying a provider or group of providers that will provide that service.

Not all service improvements and new interventions need to go through a formal procurement process ('tendering' process). An agreed 'variation of contract' may be more appropriate for some situations, for example an improvement of an existing service, or development within an integrated service. There is best practice guidance and a legal framework around procurement to ensure a fair process is adhered to.[2] Seek advice from your procurement resources and be guided as necessary. You may also need to seek procurement advice if you are unsure if there are any providers out there who can provide the service; you may have to consider how you would develop or reach the 'market'.

Contracting refers to the process of coming to an agreed contract. A contract is a formal and legally binding agreement between two or more parties. It is usually a written document. As a minimum it would include the parties involved, start date, term of the contract, services to be delivered, payment, quality requirements, governance, and contract monitoring arrangements. It may refer to an annex containing a detailed service specification.[3] Formal contracting arrangements have developed over time in the English health system (see Box 4.1).

Following any procurement and contracting steps, implementation of a new service or changes can continue through the provider.

Box 4.1 Historical note about contracting

The use of formal contracts in the NHS between an organization holding the funds (such as the Clinical Commissioning Groups in the NHS from 2013) and a hospital provider that delivers the service is relatively recent in the history of the NHS in England. In the mid-noughties, formal standard contracts between the then fundholding organizations, the Primary Care Trusts, and hospital providers were still being established and refined. The change in context as more hospitals became hospital trusts at the turn of the century rather than directly managed units of a health authority, and the movement towards a more varied provider system in the NHS at this time meant that there was an accompanying shift to 'contracts' between parties rather than the previous agreements between different aspects of the health system. Before that, the work of the key commissioning stages still needed to be done but may have resulted in a service level agreement arrangement rather than the later more formal contracts. In contrast, arrangements for the provision of general practice services and the NHS have a long history of operating through more formal contractual arrangements.

Monitoring and evaluation

At some point in the future when the service is up and running, you will need to know whether it is working as intended. You will need to monitor whether the service is meeting the outcomes and cost parameters agreed for the service.

Both monitoring and evaluation are related to assessing the situation with respect to the service goal. Monitoring deals with the progress of the here and now situation, and using information gathered to manage progress towards the goal. It is a continual process and a small number of people will be involved in doing this. Evaluation on the other hand is an intermittent process taking place at particular milestones, for example after a service has been in place for a certain period of time. It assesses whether the goal has been achieved and can involve a wide range of perspectives to do this. This process may uncover a vast array of learning which may need to be digested by all relevant stakeholders. The evaluation process may use a range of quantitative and qualitative methods. Often the best insights arise from using both.

Thus monitoring can be defined as, 'a process that follows the course of activities to help keep progress on track',[4] and evaluation can be summarized as, 'a systematic and rigorous inquiry to assess whether services or component parts achieve planned goals and analyses reasons for any discrepancy to produce information that can be used to improve its effectiveness'.

Monitoring and evaluation activities can be thought of as a range of processes including 'routine monitoring' (such as monitoring ambulance response times, or the number of clostridium difficile cases acquired in a healthcare environment); 'occasional monitoring' (such as a five-yearly oral health survey of 0 to 5 year olds); or 'intentional information seeking' (such as a service review or a specific evaluation of effectiveness).

Thinking ahead in the commissioning cycle

You will now have a better idea of the contribution of monitoring in securing effective health services. You will also have picked up that the ability to monitor relies on a couple of practical things being in place from earlier in the commissioning cycle. One of the key project management skills in commissioning is thinking ahead.

Firstly, the goals and objectives of the service that has been introduced should be clear by now, as they would have been needed for the service specification. You will not be able to monitor whether or not a service is achieving its goals if you do not know what the goals are. A goal may be, 'to make sure all people with suspected stroke in our population are assessed at a stroke centre for diagnosis'. A standard to be met might be 'all eligible people with ischaemic stroke should be offered thrombolysis within current best practice limits'. The time limits for supplying relevant information and the intervals it should be provided at should also have been clarified in the earlier specification or contract stages.

Secondly, the practicalities of collecting such monitoring information should have been clarified at earlier provider selection and implementation stages. There is little point in specifying a measure for which it is not possible to acquire the data. Measures for monitoring progress should be agreed before the start of the contract. Information collected as part of a national or other routine dataset is easier but there may be other relevant measures required. The organization providing the service will need to have a system in place to collect this information. Only then can monitoring happen when a service is up and running. Learning from monitoring and any evaluation can then be used to make ongoing refinements of the commissioning and delivery of the service.

Commissioning is a multidisciplinary effort

As Figure 4.1 infers, the business of commissioning is a multidisciplinary effort. A 'dream team' would comprise inputs from colleagues contributing a range of complementary skills, spanning commissioning management skills, population healthcare perspectives, finance, contracting, and information skills, with access to procurement, legal, and communications support. Additional specific clinical pathway knowledge can be brought in as necessary for specific pathways. Ideally each person would have some general understanding of the rationale behind the commissioning cycle components, as well as bringing in their specific inputs and resources they can access. Together the multidisciplinary effort enables the cycle (see Box 4.2).

What if we cannot start at the 'beginning' of the cycle?

When trying to use an evidence-based approach we do not always have the luxury of starting at the problem definition stage. However, do not be too deterred by this, real life can be messy. Often a service or contract is already in place, so the starting point to contribute to the cycle may be when you are assessing the service for the first time. Similarly, at the contracting stage the health outcomes associated with a contract will still need to be specified for monitoring, and of course at a prioritization and planning stage, guidance about effective interventions and opportunity costs come into play. Whatever the starting point there are always opportunities to enhance the quality of commissioning and make it more focused on health gain. Sometimes in real life, a service is in place and the outcomes to be measured are not clear, then perhaps here is an opportunity to assess against best practice outcomes e.g. through seeking assurance from providers from a clinical audit, to see how the service compares to best practice and use the

> ### Box 4.2 **Skills needed for a multidisciplinary commissioning team**
>
> - *Programme and project management skills:* to manage the overall commissioning process, build the service specification, and engage the market as necessary. Ideally have an overall strategic fit perspective as well as project viewpoint.
> - *Population healthcare skills:* to include advice about amenable health needs, advice about outcomes and quality measures to be monitored, and a population outcome perspective to the prioritization process.
> - *Information and finance:* to support the financial and quality monitoring of the contract and evaluation of the service.
> - *Specific knowledge of the health pathway of interest.*
> - *Procurement and contracting skills:* to advise on the procurement processes if necessary and advise on legal matters of contracting.
> - *Communications and administrative* support if not already part of the commissioning management support team. To communicate about the process to stakeholders, co-ordinate lay member representation, and public engagement as necessary.

learning from that for the next commissioning cycle. Basically, do not be afraid to apply evidence-based principles, whatever the starting point in the commissioning cycle you find yourself in with your service of interest. Box 4.3 is a short exercise to familiarize with how real-life questions in commissioning can connect with the cycle.

New structures, same population health gain goals

As you will have gathered by now, the overall goal of achieving population health gain from health services decision-making and its related commissioning processes remains pertinent whatever the commissioning and delivery structures of the day.

Box 4.3 **Exercise: Commissioning cycle questions**

The following questions are useful to consider in day-to-day commissioning work. They are related to the commissioning cycle (problem definition, planning and prioritization, contracting and procurement, and monitoring and evaluation). Can you work out which parts of the cycle most directly relate to each one? A 'commissioner' in this context is anyone working in a health or care commissioning organization who contributes directly or indirectly to the commissioning cycle processes.

  (i) How good is the evidence of the problem?
 (ii) What are the effective things worth doing?
(iii) What data do I need to understand the picture? (Size of the problem, who is affected? Is there an effective practical intervention? What is the size of the health benefit and for how many people? What is the cost overall and cost-effectiveness? What services already exist to serve this need?)
 (iv) How to make priority setting decisions in a consistent and transparent manner? In a way that opportunity costs are clear.
  (v) What is effective, cost-effective, *and* affordable?
 (vi) What measures should be spelt out in the quality schedule?
(vii) How do I follow the correct procedures for procurement?
(viii) How does this process contribute to reducing health inequalities?
 (ix) How well does the service work in practice in our patch?
  (x) What mechanisms do we have to feedback and improve the quality of services commissioned?

Answers: D = Problem definition, P = Prioritization and planning, CP = Contracting and procurement, ME = Monitoring and evaluation.
(i) D (ii) D (iii) D (iv) P (v) P (vi) CP (vii) CP (viii) D, P, CP, and ME (ix) ME (x) ME.

A system that distinguishes between commissioners and providers places greater onus on the commissioner for ensuring there are plans in place that lead to population health gain. This was the landscape of the NHS in England after the legislation bringing in the 'purchaser–provider split' of the early 1990s,[5,6] and that continued to develop with various reshapings of the local commissioning layer infrastructure and initiatives throughout the noughties.[7] This further continued with the substantial reshaping of local commissioning infrastructure following the Health and Social Care Act 2012.[8] How successful the commissioner was at achieving it is a different matter, but the balance of responsibility for improving population health through health services did fall on those commissioning for populations to oversee. Leading up to 1990, the local health authorities of the time had responsibilities for both the planning and provision of local services, with hospitals being in effect directly managed units of the regional tier of health authorities, and primary care services (e.g. GP services) were secured from primary care contractors through local NHS committees. Thus those in charge of planning services and those in charge of delivering the services were both operating in a system connected through a common regional tier which in theory oversaw both. The future may, or may not, bring those planning services and those in charge of delivering services closer again, and with new added features perhaps, such as blending in aspects of social care (for example the development of integrated care systems, see Box 4.4). As with any truly universal system, with whole population coverage providing a comprehensive range of services, the routes of public accountability and governance for new models will have to be properly scrutinized to make sure that equitable access according to need and population coverage remain fundamental principles. However none of these variants materially changes the need for those holding the resources to plan effectively how best to meet the needs of the population. The principles of a population approach to securing services and decision-making continue to apply.

Ready to try

Finally just be aware that the work related to the different stages of a commissioning cycle can often be highly relevant even if it is not labelled as 'commissioning cycle' work as such. You will recognise that much ongoing service redesign and development work does not start from scratch at the beginning of a squeaky clean cycle. That need not be a problem in practice, the key things about being clear about the goals of a service, what measures to monitor and evaluate, and having a population approach are still highly relevant.

Box 4.4 **Integrated organizations and integrated care systems**

Integrated care providers (ICP) are essentially a collaboration of providers for a population. It is a means of organizing services that tries to overcome some of the disjointedness that patients may experience as a result of a care journey involving several different providers. There are various ways of trying to do this. Collaboration can be 'horizontal', across general practice and community-based health services, or 'vertical', across general practice, community health, and hospital services. In theory the models could also include social care, public health services, and mental health services components. An ambitious model of integrated provision would include both horizontal and vertical integration, and social care, public health services, and mental health services. Even more ambitious models of integrated provision might include all of those elements, and take on some responsibility for whole population planning.

The term integrated care system (ICS) has been used to describe the overall arrangement of key providers in a population system (whether organized into ICP entities or not) along with all the other commissioning elements of running a population healthcare system on that footprint.[9] In theory if this is used as a standard approach throughout health services in England, the aggregate coverage of all the ICSs would need to cover the whole England population.

What are the goals of an integrated system?
Various goals have been put forward and include;

- to improve patient experience, coordination, and quality of care;
- to control expenditure;
- using it as a means of integrating health and social care;
- to increase collective responsibility across the system of commissioners and providers for financial performance and health outcomes.

Would ICPs bring provision and commissioning expertise closer?

Essentially an ICP is about a group of providers working together with closer coordination under a single umbrella (in theory a single provider could also discharge all this), at the same time working closely with the local health service commissioner(s) for a population. In theory such arrangements would shift the providers' balance of focus from treatment and care of individuals to also include management of the pre-illness health of a population whilst working within a cash-limited budget. That is, provider organizations begin to take on a population commissioning perspective.

What do we know about their effectiveness so far?

At the time of writing, much evidence about the effectiveness of such integrated structures has yet to be gathered. The effectiveness on improving quality is mixed,[10,11] and the impact on healthcare spending remains unclear.[10,12]

Questions remaining include:

- How effective is the ICP type model at providing a comprehensive service? That is, the provision of preventive, primary, secondary, community, and mental health care and possibly social care as well, as opposed to a more limited product range?
- Can integrated systems reduce use of healthcare services and therefore healthcare costs?
- Can integrated systems improve quality of care within the overall budget?

Reflection

Think about a service you are working on or would like to work on. What monitoring would you put in place to check your plans are on track to deliver the health outcomes you are aiming for?

Consider the work of your colleagues. Which parts of the cycle does their work contribute to?

References

1. Gray JAM. *Evidence-based healthcare. How to make health policy and management decisions.* Churchill Livingstone, 2001.
2. Monitor. Procurement, choice and competition in the NHS: documents and guidance. Available at: https://www.gov.uk/government/collections/procurement-choice-and-competition-in-the-nhs-documents-and-guidance
3. NHS England. NHS Standard Contract: 2017/19 to 2018/19. May 2018. Available at: https://www.england.nhs.uk/nhs-standard-contract/2017-19-update-may/
4. St Leger S, Schneiden H, Walsworth-Bell JP. *Evaluating health services effectiveness: guide for health professionals, service managers and policy makers.* Open University Press, 1991.
5. Department for Health and Social Security, HMSO. Working for patients. 1989.
6. HMSO. National Health Service and Community Care Act 1990.
7. Department of Health. Shifting the balance of power within the NHS. July 2001.
8. HMSO. Health and Social Care Act 2012.
9. NHS England. The NHS Long Term Plan. January 2019.
10. Baxter S, Johnson M, Chambers D, Sutton A, Goyder E, Booth A. The effects of integrated care: a systematic review of UK and international evidence. *BMC Health Serv Res* 2018;18(1):350. doi:10.1186/s12913-018-3161-3
11. National Audit Office. Developing new care models through NHS Vanguards, HC129. June 2018. Available at: https://www.nao.org.uk/wp-content/uploads/2018/06/Developing-new-care-models-through-NHS-Vanguards.pdf
12. Iacobucci G. 'No compelling evidence' shows that integrated care in England saves money, says NAO. *BMJ* 2017;356:j704.

5
Public Health

Three Key Domains

You will have seen in previous chapters that a population approach is an integral part of healthcare commissioning and that this focus of work is recognized within public health practice as Healthcare Public Health.

This is just one of the three domains of public health practice. This chapter is an orientation about these three core domains of public health practice, to provide further context about these aspects of an overall health system. You will have gathered by now that working effectively in a population healthcare system involves being 'multilingual' to some extent. That is to say that in your work or studies you are likely to come across various 'health service speak' and 'general management speak', as well as the language of other agencies and disciplines. Assimilating this is not as daunting as it sounds, but it does require an openness about contributions from different disciplines and to ask questions as needed. So here is a little context from the public health arena to add to your repertoire so that you can enjoy engaging in these topics with confidence and clarity.

Main points to be familiar with . . .

- The three core domains of public health practice.
- In a healthcare system you will interact with all three aspects.
- One of these domains is directly relevant to the commissioning of health services. This 'healthcare public health' component is concerned with improving health outcomes through health services quality and effectiveness. It is an integral part of the commissioning cycle for health services.

Commissioning and a Population Approach to Health Services Decision-Making. Julie Sin, Oxford University Press (2020). © Oxford University Press. DOI: 10.1093/oso/9780198840732.001.0001

Health status of populations

In contrast to the individual picture of health status presented at the patient–clinician level, public health practice is concerned with the health status of populations and amenable ways to improve and protect that. That is, in public health practice, the 'patient' as such is the population (recognizing that interactions at the individual level aggregate up to population outcomes). Effectiveness is thus considered at the population level, as well as recognizing the importance of effective individual interactions.

Terminology and definitions

Public health is a commonly heard term in health services and public discourse, though without specific clarification its use can mean many different things to different people in different situations and this can sometimes wrong-foot discussions. For example, when cited, is it being used to refer to a health improvement focus, or to communicable disease control, or a particular group of health services deemed public health, or to a multi-agency approach, or to a societal approach in general, or the effectiveness of health services at a population level, or to health information knowledge, or is it a nod to the overarching notion of prevention, or indeed to something else? Whilst such a broad and unspecified use of the term may be sufficient in some circumstances, sometimes it is more useful to have greater clarity about why the term is being used in that situation.

It is worth being aware that in the general use of the term, there is the wider societal objective of public health which refers to the broad engagement of all relevant parts of society and public systems for better health in the population, and there is also the use of the term public health referring to the work of public health and its staff as a branch of practice within a health and care system. If you feel that a discussion would benefit from acknowledging these distinctions, make the distinction clear to enable your discussions.

Public health has classically been described as, 'the science and art of preventing disease, prolonging life and promoting health through the organised efforts of society' by Acheson.[1] This remains a resonant and useful high-level definition, which particularly captures the societal objective. It recognizes the vast context in which health outcomes are shaped whilst recognizing that there are many contributory parts to the effort. It is also versatile enough to cope with changes in emphasis over time of different burdens of disease in the population (e.g. from the dominance of living environment causes and acute infectious diseases of the past to chronic diseases and emerging conditions of the present).

Three domains of public health

In practical terms, public health practice covers three core domains of practice in England.[2,3,4] They are shown diagrammatically in Figure 5.1. Together they aim to protect health or improve population health outcomes. They are complementary and reinforcing through different opportunities in the healthcare and wider environment. Their 'entry points' into tackling health issues from a population perspective span the full chronology of a health condition and its impacts.

These domains are:

1. *Health Improvement.* This looks upstream at predisposing factors and modifiable causes of health conditions.
2. *Health Protection.* This domain deals with acute threats to the health status of the population as we know it.
3. *Healthcare Public Health.* This aspect is concerned with the condition in-hand and the service opportunities for effective care and improving outcomes.

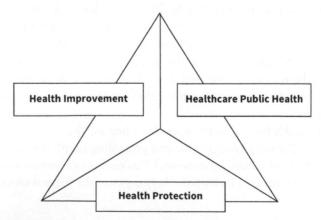

Figure 5.1 Three domains of public health practice

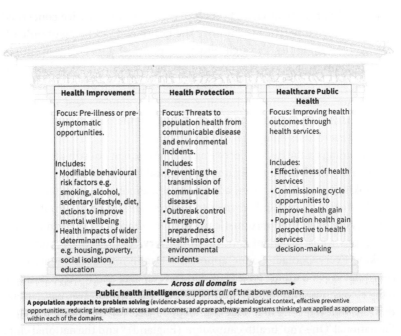

Figure 5.2 Three domains ('Pillars') of public health and underpinning approaches

It is worth being familiar with these terms so you can work out how they might fit with your issue in-hand (or not), and have more meaningful conversations about what effectively can be done with the resources available within your local system. All domains involve both technical and leadership skills as relevant to the situation. The three domains can also be usefully presented as three 'pillars of public health'. All are supported by public health intelligence (the use of information to support achievement of health outcomes at a population level) and a population approach to problem-solving (see Figure 5.2). The domains are a practical grouping of the population health challenges to be tackled and the opportunities to face them. Let's look at these domains briefly in turn.

The work of Health Improvement

Also known as health promotion and wider determinants work. This deals with opportunities for improving health *before* the onset or detection of illness.

Health improvement is the branch of public health practice concerned with policies and practice to improve the health and wellbeing of individuals and communities through efforts to promote and enable healthier lifestyle choices. It also acknowledges and addresses, where feasible, underlying socioeconomic and environmental impacts on population health from factors such as poverty, housing, education, employment, etc. (wider determinants of health). It can be thought of as the part of public health practice that focuses on upstream prevention.

Depending on the issue, effective action may be best coordinated at a national or a more local level. Examples at a local level include the provision of smoking cessation services, advice about alcohol consumption, weight management services, and services to reduce social isolation. Another example is the offer of opportunistic prevention advice for common chronic conditions whilst a patient is in receipt of services for other reasons, the 'Making Every Contact Count' approach.[5] Health improvement activities coordinated at a national level would include alcohol and tobacco duties to reduce consumption, minimum unit pricing for alcohol, seat belt legislation, awareness raising to reduce overall population disease burden such as the national 'One You' health campaigns (England),[6] and the national child measurement programme.[7]

The work of Health Protection

Health protection is the branch of public health concerned with policies and practice to improve the prevention and control of communicable diseases (infectious diseases) and environmental threats to the health of the population.

It provides advice about health protection matters to the healthcare system and the wider community. It leads on communicable disease outbreaks and their control. It can be thought of as the 'blue light' emergency response part of public health practice (although as with other blue light responding agencies such as fire and police services, there is also a strong preventive focus as well, e.g. infection control and immunizations in the case of health protection). For detail on specific practices and scenario handling there are dedicated resources on communicable disease control and the domain overall.[8,9]

Depending on the system of the day, this health protection resource may be nationally arranged but situated on a regional or sub-regional basis to support smaller localities as needed,[12] or situated within smaller local geographies as a health protection resource (as with some previous models of health protection).

Specific aspects of health protection include:

- surveillance and monitoring of infectious diseases;
- outbreak control;
- contact tracing;
- immunization programmes;
- emergency planning and training for incidents;
- health impacts of chemical, radiological, and biological hazards.

The work of Healthcare Public Health (HCPH)

Healthcare public health (sometimes called health services improvement domain) is the branch of public health concerned with policies and practice to improve health outcomes for the population through the effectiveness and quality of health services. It is part of the essential behind-the-scenes work of commissioning health services for the population. It is possibly the least well-articulated domain of public health practice outside of the health services sphere, though it is a highly relevant perspective to health services commissioning and decision-making. In addition, because its practice is also a branch of the public health family, when present in NHS commissioning it also enables links to other specialist public health advice if needed.

As with all domains of public health practice, its contributions to the health system encompasses both leadership and technical contributions. Below is a working definition:

Healthcare Public Health is the branch of public health practice and a synergistic part of health services commissioning (or equivalent processes to secure health services) that relates to the skills, activities, and leadership to enable population health gain through the commissioning and provision of services.

Healthcare public health and the commissioning system

As HCPH is concerned with improving outcomes through effective health services, this usually means working within the commissioning processes (or other equivalent strategic planning process if there is no commissioner–provider split). And conversely, a multidisciplinary approach to commissioning would include support and advice from HCPH resources.[10,11] Examples of HCPH work at the strategy and governance level include population health gain inputs to:

- health services decision-making at board or governing body level;
- policy making and guidance e.g. for clinical networks, medicines management, and commissioning in general;
- quality and performance information, interpretation, and decision-making;
- development of prioritization frameworks and decision-making processes to incorporate health gain as a criteria.

Examples of HCPH work at a day-to-day business level include population health gain perspective to the review and redesign of pathways, with respect to:

- outcomes to measure and framing questions about healthcare needs;
- access criteria and care-pathway coherence;
- effective opportunities and cost-effectiveness;
- interpretation of population-level information and advice about evaluation of services.

A blend of these governance and technical perspectives can also be applied to individual funding request considerations. Also as part of a local system's leadership efforts, HCPH supports the multidisciplinary commissioning system as a matter of course and contributes to building capacity for these skills in the system.

Healthcare public health at provider organizations

In the provider setting, healthcare public health skills can contribute to healthcare quality or effectiveness work, for example through evaluation of services, audit, and providing a population perspective to strategic discussions.

A working appreciation of the aims of the commissioning cycle is also relevant from the provider perspective. For example, the leadership level of any provider organization would need to have an understanding of the needs of the local population, relevant outcomes to measure in order to monitor service quality, and an awareness of the overall patient pathways and interdependencies for the population it serves.

A word about prevention

Although one of the public health domains clearly focuses on early preventive opportunities at the population level (health improvement), it is important to remember that all the domains recognize this principle, and indeed many disciplines in the health and care field have a preventive aspect to their core work at the individual patient level. An example would be the GP identifying and managing a patient's high blood pressure or type 2 diabetes to reduce longer term complications. Also as part of the general care of the patient, a clinician would advise about the impact of modifiable risk factors such as tobacco smoking, alcohol intake, and weight, if these factors were identified within the history and examination. They can let patients know about further services as appropriate or advise and manage directly. Similarly, hospitals may have an active strategy to reduce modifiable risk factors for the population of patients it serves. Examples include opportunistically identifying patients who could benefit from lifestyle risk factor modifications advice (a 'Making Every Contact Count' approach), using a 'smoke free' hospital policy, offering help to pregnant women to stop smoking from specialist stop smoking services, and linking patients with an alcohol-related admission to alcohol liaison services. Hospitals may also have specific prevention processes as part of their patients' general care e.g. falls prevention protocols and pressure ulcer prevention. The 'Making Every Contact Count' approach can also be used in the wider community with respect to people in contact with social care and other professionals in the community. Thus the task of prevention is not the job of a single discipline but the proper interplay of all relevant parts of the system.

Public health commissioned services

As a result of the Health and Social Care Act 2012, certain health services were grouped as 'public health commissioned services' in England (such as sexual health services, child measurement programme, school nursing) and monies were ring-fenced to be administered by newly formed local authority public health departments.[13] This meant that the new local public health departments had direct commissioning responsibility for such health services (see Box 5.1). (At the time of writing that accountability model is still in place, though in some areas those health services might also be part of a wider health and social care commissioning system). The core work involved in commissioning these services is essentially the commissioning cycle and this is not unlike the commissioning of any other health service. As such they are best considered as a range of health services that need to be commissioned, subject to all the principles of any other type of health services commissioning, regardless of the organizational route that the funding flows down.

Box 5.1 Public health in the English health system as part of the 2012 Act

In the English health system, leading up to the implementation of the Health and Social Care Act 2012,[14] the fundholding organization of local health services (the commissioner) was the Primary Care Trust (PCT). These PCTs oversaw commissioning of a comprehensive range of health services. The 2012 Act led to the separation of the then NHS commissioning functions into local Clinical Commissioning Groups and regional NHS England components and also dispersed the local public health functions into new organizational bases. For orientation and in the spirit of enabling 'multilingualism' for coherent discussions about health services, the three emergent 'homes' for public health functions following the 2012 Act are described.

The most prominent of these new public health homes was **Public Health England (PHE)**,[12] a national arrangement (an executive arm of the Department of Health) with regional outposts. The main public health function delivered and led from here being health protection expertise to deal with communicable disease and environmental threats to health. PHE also oversee the production and release of a wide range of population health information. Over time some PHE areas have developed arm's length support to local authority public health teams in the health improvement and healthcare public health arenas as well.

Notably, although PHE may have a degree of influence, it has little formal authority over the decisions of the local authorities, including their local decisions about public health.

A chunk of the local public health functions would reside with the new **NHS England** after the 2012 Act.[15] These were mainly population screening programmes and immunization programmes (such as childhood immunizations and 'flu vaccinations) and some healthcare public health support to specialized services.[16]

And finally, the remainder of the local public health functions were to reside with local authorities (upper tier and unitary level). These **local authority public health departments** would receive a ring-fenced budget to secure a set of mandatory public health services for the local area. Examples of these services were, 'NHS Health checks', sexual health services, child measurement service, and school nursing. Local public health departments also had to ensure there were robust health protection arrangements for the population, provide local NHS commissioners with advice about effectiveness and health outcomes, and work with other council departments on health improvement issues.[17] These local public health departments would be accountable to their respective local authorities. As local authorities are local statutory bodies, there is no formal accountability of the local authorities to the national PHE system, aside from through the ring-fenced grant, though locally there may be working relationships.

Funding for these public health functions originate from the Department of Health. In 2013–14 spending on public health functions nationally was estimated to be £5.8 billion,[17] and Department of Health spending overall was £106.5 billion.[18]

Reflection

Do you know where the different public health teams are located in your local health system?

When you last had a public health type question, which aspect(s) did you wish to consider specifically?

References

1. Acheson D. Public health in England. The report of the committee of inquiry into the future development of the public health function. HMSO, 1988.
2. Griffiths S, Jewell T, Donnelly P. Public health in practice: the three domains of public health. *Public Health* 2005;119(10):907–913.
3. House of Commons. House of Commons Health Committee, Public health post-2013. Second report of session 2016-17 HC 140. July 2016.
4. Faculty of Public Health. Good Public Health Practice Framework 2016. Available at: https://www.fph.org.uk/media/1304/good-public-health-practice-framework_-2016_final.pdf
5. Health Education England. Making Every Contact Count. Available at: https://www.makingeverycontactcount.co.uk/
6. Public Health England. About One You. Available at: https://www.nhs.uk/oneyou/about-one-you/
7. NHS Digital. National child measurement programme. October 2017. Available at: https://files.digital.nhs.uk/publication/j/n/nati-chil-meas-prog-eng-2016-2017-rep.pdf
8. Public Health England. Health protection. Available at: https://www.gov.uk/topic/health-protection
9. Ghebrehewet S, Samuel AG, Baxter D, Shears P, Conrad D, Kliner M. *Health Protection*. Oxford University Press, 2016.
10. Department of Health. Healthcare public health advice to clinical commissioning groups. Gateway reference 17804. June 2012.
11. PHE publications. Core Offer: The Healthcare Public Health Advice Service to Clinical Commissioning Groups. Gateway number 2017228. August 2017.
12. Public Health England. PHE regions, local centres and emergency contacts. Available at: https://www.gov.uk/government/collections/contacts-public-health-england-regions-local-centres-and-emergency
13. Department of Health. Public health ring-fenced grant conditions-2014/15, Local Authority Circular. December 2013. Available at: https://assets.publishing.service.gov.uk/government/uploads/system/uploads/attachment_data/file/269464/local_authority_circular_dh_2013_3_a.pdf
14. HMSO. Health and Social Care Act 2012.
15. Department of Health. Public health functions to be exercised by the NHS Commissioning Board. Gateway reference 18035. November 2012. Available at: https://www.gov.uk/government/uploads/system/uploads/attachment_data/file/213153/s7A-master-131114-final.pdf
16. Department of Health. NHS public health functions agreement 2017-2018. Public health functions to be exercised by NHS England. Gateway Reference 06336. NHS England Publications, March 2014.
17. National Audit Office. Public Health England's Grant to Local Authorities. 2014. Available at: https://www.nao.org.uk/wp-content/uploads/2014/12/Public-health-england's-grant-to-local-authorities.pdf
18. Department of Health. Annual report and accounts 2013-14. HC14. 2014.

6

Evidence Hierarchy

Evidence of what works, to what extent it might work, and under what conditions, is an important part of the knowledge we need to make decisions. To make use of such evidence, we need to know what we are dealing with before we can use the available evidence to inform decisions.

For decision-making we are often faced with the question, 'how likely will this work?' or 'how strong is the evidence for this?', or at least the questions should occur to us. Even if you have a report in front of you covering the exact topic you need, how much should you trust its findings and how do the methods used stand up to scrutiny? It will help to have some bearings and an 'evidence hierarchy' to help deal with the basic question of 'how reliable is this evidence?'

Some study methods are considered to be more reliable than others for discerning the strength of the relationship between cause and effect. For orientation and ease of use, an adapted ABCD categorization system is offered in this chapter, based on classic evidence hierarchies from the research literature. It can be applied to many types of papers and articles that one might come across during everyday work. It can be used by anyone regardless of professional background.

Main points to be familiar with . . .

- An evidence hierarchy is an explicit guide indicating the degree of robustness of the evidence gathering method used to discern cause and effect.
- Have a basic evidence hierarchy you can apply with ease to the material you come across, particularly in situations about proposed interventions.
- Be able to spot the study types.

Commissioning and a Population Approach to Health Services Decision-Making. Julie Sin, Oxford University Press (2020). © Oxford University Press. DOI: 10.1093/oso/9780198840732.001.0001

The concept of an evidence hierarchy

Essentially, some study designs are less open to bias than others in trying to understand true effects. A bias is any systematic error (i.e. not a random error) that leads to a mistaken estimation of the true effect. It can result from trends in data collection, analysis, interpretation, and publication that systematically lead to a conclusion that is different from the true effect. Evidence from some studies is more prone to biases because of the manner in which information is gathered. That is not to say such information cannot be considered during decision-making but it does help if we are aware of what we are dealing with. Applying an evidence hierarchy helps to make the reliability of the evidence more explicit whether it shows positive or negative findings. An evidence hierarchy is essentially a rule of thumb grading system in which those study designs and methods which are less open to biases are ranked higher than those based on methods more prone to biases. It is primarily used for assessing studies of cause and effect.

Useful situations

An evidence hierarchy is useful when:

- assessing briefing or policy material;
- assessing the merits of (the evidence component) of a business case for service improvement;
- compiling a business case;
- reading a journal article;
- taking part in prioritization or decision-making work.

Often the task in hand will not be labelled as requiring an evidence hierarchy approach, but it will still be highly relevant to use it. You will find yourself in these situations quite regularly if you watch out for them. For example when reviewing reports for a discussion, or even gauging whether evidence during a conversation is drawing on significant evidence or anecdote.

A basic system for assessing cause and effect

The principles of an evidence hierarchy have been observed for some decades in the health and healthcare sphere. The Canadian Task Force for Preventive Health Care originally described the use of such an approach for assessing health interventions and there have been many other working versions with a similar rationale over time.[1,2,3] From such origins work has since evolved with using this level of evidence approach to align more directly with the task of making recommendations for practice,[4] though the basic approach remains worth understanding in itself and is helpful in making sense of ongoing developments in this arena. Initially such tools were used to assess interventions in the clinical setting but there is no reason why the principles cannot be applied to any research evidence purporting to establish cause and effect.

There can be more detailed sub-levels within each level of a grading system but the basic trend in an evidence hierarchy is the same. A basic evidence hierarchy would look like Table 6.1.

Table 6.1 A basic evidence hierarchy

Evidence type (based on design)	The highest level of evidence showing the effect of interest is based on at least one well-conducted ...
A	Aggregate analysis of relevant randomized controlled trials: **Meta-analysis** and **systematic review** or, **Randomized controlled trial**
B	Observational study with a comparison group: **Cohort study** **Case-control study** or, 'natural experiments' where there is a clear relevant comparison group.
C	Observational study with no comparison group: **Cross-sectional surveys** **Case-series** and **case-reports**
D	**Expert consensus** and **reports** without any of the above.

Note: Where there are doubts about the quality of the study, despite the purported study design given, drop to a level below.

As you can see, the link between cause and effect is more open to bias as we move from A towards D in the chart. The randomized controlled trial (RCT) design is not difficult to spot if present. Essentially in this type of design study participants are randomized to an active intervention group or to a comparison group that does not receive the intervention being studied (a control group). Ideally both the study participants and the investigators administering the trial are unaware of which group participants are in until the trial has finished ('double blinded' trial). The aim is for all groups to be treated identically except for the intervention being studied. This type of study is commonly used to assess the effectiveness of drug treatments for example. Type B evidence in the hierarchy refers to observational studies with a comparison group. These can still be highly analytical in design but no active interventions are delivered as such. Inferences about cause and effect are drawn by comparing the preceding risk factors of those with the disease with those without the disease. Cohort studies and case-control studies are the main types in this group. Type C evidence is again descriptive and observational in nature but set up without a comparison group. Whilst their ability to discern cause and effect is lower than evidence types higher up in the hierarchy, these studies can contribute to generating new insights and hypotheses about conditions. Type D evidence would cover opinions of respected authorities without a clear basis drawn from higher levels. With any topic you are looking for the highest level of evidence to address your key question.

The hierarchy helps to understand the robustness of the methods used to answer the (cause and effect) question it set out to address. It is a guide to the degree of confidence and caution you should have in its findings. It will be the direction that the overall body of knowledge in this area is pointing to that is important, not just a single primary study. Indeed the ongoing development of methods to grade evidence in the guideline development sphere has emphasized assessing the evidence overall for a particular outcome rather than just on grading individual studies (though assessing the robustness of each study remains part of that effort). It has also been made clearer for guideline producers that certain factors can strengthen the reliability of the overall findings (e.g. a dose-response effect) and certain factors can reduce their reliability (e.g. risk of bias, inconsistency, and indirectness). Many guideline-generating authorities have adopted an internationally recognized grading methodology (GRADE system)[4,5] to help assess the strength of the recommendations they produce.[6,7,8]

From the day-to-day commissioning perspective, where the practitioner is faced on a daily basis with a number of reports and types of evidence, from many different sources spanning a variety of subjects, being familiar with the concept of a levels of evidence approach to study designs relating to cause and effect, and being able to gauge the quality of individual reports and the evidence they offer per se remains a useful part of the practical armoury of a commissioner.

You will need to be able to spot the main study types that assess effectiveness of health services or cause and effect. The following section describes the study types in more detail for further understanding and to help you spot them with ease.

Spotting the different study types

Systematic reviews and meta-analyses

A systematic review is a review of a collection of primary research studies that have used explicit and reproducible methods. This evidence type enables large amounts of information to be assimilated quickly by decision-makers in the health service and by policy makers. The findings of many studies are systematically compiled into a single analysis. Explicit methods are used to identify and reject studies for inclusion and in theory the conclusions are more reliable because of the larger amount of relevant data the analysis can draw upon.

A quantitative systematic review is a meta-analysis. This is a mathematical synthesis of the results of two or more primary studies that addressed the same hypothesis in the same way. This increases the precision of the overall result. Usually meta-analyses are conducted on randomized control trials. There are recognized good practice standard methods for conducting systematic reviews and meta-analysis.[9]

It is helpful if the meta-analysis discusses the following points to help the reader make sense of its results:

• Publication bias. This particular bias can affect meta-analysis results and arises when studies with positive results have been more likely to have been published than those with negative results so the aggregate effect overestimates the true effect. The potential for publication bias should be assessed.

- Heterogeneity or variability of studies. For a meaningful summary, meta-analysis should only be conducted when a group of studies is sufficiently similar (homogeneous) in terms of the subjects involved, interventions, and outcomes to be measured. Combining studies that differ substantially can yield a meaningless overall result. The presence of heterogeneity, or not, should be discussed.[9] Whilst it might not be possible to have a meaningful combined result if heterogeneity is present, examination of the reasons for the variability among studies can lead to useful insights that can be used to plan care and understand different practical aspects that may have a bearing on the situation (for example differences in the setting or the way the intervention was delivered).

- Sensitivity analysis may also be offered as part of a meta-analysis. This looks at what happens if the meta-analysis were analysed slightly differently, e.g. if different arbitrary age cut-off points were used, to test if the findings are still robust.

Randomized controlled trials

Randomized controlled trials (RCT) test the effectiveness of specific interventions (e.g. drug or therapeutic procedure) under controlled conditions. Conducted well, they provide a rigorous means of assessing cause and effect.

Study participants are assigned to an intervention or control group by random allocation to ensure there are no systematic baseline differences between the groups. The intervention group receive the drug, therapy, or mode of service delivery that is being tested. The control group(s) receive a standard therapy or placebo. Ideally both the participants and the investigators administering the trial do not know which arm of the trial the participants are in. This double blinding ensures that any preconceived views of subjects and clinicians cannot bias the assessment of outcomes. If only the participant is unaware of the arm of the trial they are in then it is a single blinded trial.

These rigorous measures help ensure all participants are treated identically apart from the intervention under study. The outcomes of interest, for example disease remission or prevention of onset of disease, is compared between groups to assess the effectiveness of the intervention compared to control. Multi-centred RCTs increase the study sample size and can also improve the generalizability of findings.

RCT studies are more common in the clinical trial setting and are rarer in the field of non-clinical setting interventions, where practicalities such as blinding, or a long time lag between cause and effect may mean an RCT design is not appropriate. For example it is impractical to be 'blind' to some interventions like physical activity though different levels of activity could be compared.

Things to watch out for with RCTs are the duration of follow-up and whether 'intention to treat' analysis is used. As regards follow-up, it should be long enough to be meaningful in real-life, for example follow-up for say three months to study survival after treatment for acute heart attack. If 'intention to treat' analysis is used, participants that have dropped out during the study are still included in the analysis to avoid attrition bias affecting the result (that is when those that have dropped out are different in some way to those that do not drop out).

Also on reviewing the findings of such a study ask yourself whether there is enough information to understand the benefits of the new treatment in absolute terms as well as in relative terms. For example a treatment with 15% risk reduction (a relative statistic) of an adverse outcome when the risk of the unwanted outcome is very low, would benefit far less people in absolute terms compared to a 15% risk reduction where the risk of the unwanted outcome is very high in the population. There are other factors to be taken into account as well and it does not mean the former situation is not worth considering, but the absolute numbers must also be understood alongside any relative statistics in reporting.

Well known examples of RCTs are the ISIS trials (International Studies of Infarct Survival). These were large multi-centred RCTs conducted over 1981 to 1993.[10,11,12,13] They examined and demonstrated the effectiveness of thrombolysis (clot-dissolving drugs) and other prevention therapies to improve survival in people with acute myocardial infarction (heart attack). Overall learning from these studies and others eventually paved the way to wider introduction of thrombolysis and standards of treatment for acute myocardial infarction.

Cohort studies

A cohort study is a type of observational study to understand risk factors for disease (or other outcomes of interest). They contribute knowledge about cause and effect. A cohort of people without the disease of interest is followed-up over time, noting any potential risk factors (as far as one can glean at that point) to assess whether certain risk factors increase the chance of developing a particular condition. This type of study may take many years to conclude.

The incidence rates between different sub-groups of the study population who have developed the disease are compared with the subgroup who have not developed the disease, with respect to different levels of exposure to a risk factor that is under investigation (e.g. environmental toxin, drug exposure, or another risk factor).

Whilst cohort studies cannot show causation, they are useful for yielding information about risk factors for disease. They can also provide information about incidence (the number of new cases per year). Such studies are however time and resource consuming to conduct and this has to be taken into account. A large population is observed, usually for many years as this can be the time it takes for the disease of interest to develop e.g. coronary heart disease or cancers. Some losses to follow up are probably inevitable and the impact of this, or not should be included in the discussion of results.

A well-known example is the cohort study of British civil servants initiated in 1967,[14] which described an inverse relationship between employment grade and mortality from coronary heart disease. A second related cohort study, the Whitehall II study, continued to examine this.[15] As well as beginning to put a spotlight on the relationship between social and economic factors and health, these studies highlighted the need to look more closely at socioeconomic and psychosocial stressors to health, as well as traditional cardiovascular risk factors for coronary heart disease.

Case-control studies

This is another type of observational study to understand risk factors for disease. A case-control study compares a group of people who have developed a disease (or other outcome of interest) with a comparison group of people without the outcome. It looks back at the past history of exposure to a suspected risk factor and this is compared between the 'cases' and 'controls'.

Cases have developed the outcome of interest. Controls do not have the outcome and are selected from the same source population that produced the cases. They should be selected independently of whether they have been exposed to the purported risk factors or not.

As with cohort studies, case-control studies can provide important information about disease causation. However, case-control studies are quicker and less resource intensive to conduct. (Whereas a prospectively conducted cohort study has to wait for cases to become apparent in the population to then study the risk factors leading up to this, a case-control study design can be conducted more quickly as it can be instigated at the starting point of cases being apparent, and appropriate controls to compare with can be selected.) The case-control design is useful for rarer outcomes, for example some neurological diseases, and those with long latency periods between exposure and disease.

Limitations with this study type include potential inaccuracy of information recalled about levels of past exposure (recall bias); it is not suitable for rare exposures and incidence cannot be calculated.

A famous example is the case-control study by Doll and Hill in 1950[16] showing the association between tobacco smoking and carcinoma of the lung (the commonest type of lung cancer). Although the strong association could not be shown to be causal with this study type, a subsequent cohort study which was started the year after[17,18] confirmed the findings from the powerful initial case-control study.

Descriptive–non analytical studies

These include cross-sectional studies, case series, and case reports. Cross-sectional studies or surveys gather data at a point in time, for example surveys about dietary intake or physical activity in the population. They are useful for estimating prevalence and can provide insights for further investigation, but they do not test cause and effect. Information from case series and case reports can also provide an early source of new observations that could be investigated further. Whilst these methods can raise hypotheses and associations to be further investigated, they cannot estimate cause and effect. These types of evidence cannot control for biases and confounding factors in the study design.

Memorable examples of case reports were the initial reports of five cases of unusual pneumonias[19] and eight cases of Kaposi's sarcoma[20] in 1981 in previously healthy young homosexual men which alerted the scientific community about an emerging immunodeficiency condition, later known as Acquired Immunodeficiency Syndrome (HIV/AIDS).

Expert consensus

In the absence of any of the other evidence types from the hierarchy, professional consensus may the highest level of evidence you have. It may come from an expert committee or a respected professional body. This level of evidence can be awareness raising and a starting point for further research, data collection, and associated clinical improvement. However, evidence based on opinion alone cannot control for biases and confounding factors and needs to be interpreted with that understanding.

So that is a working orientation of the different study types of an evidence hierarchy to help make sense of the research evidence you might come across. The conduct and design of such studies belong to a body of methods from epidemiology and there are dedicated texts on study designs which can be consulted for more details as necessary. As a commissioner your focus is to gain confidence in interpreting and making sense of findings for your real-life context.

Different knowledge for different questions

You may have noticed that study designs at the top end of the hierarchy directly assess cause and effect whilst those nearer the bottom are hypothesis generating. This is why the hierarchy is useful for looking at the robustness of study designs for assessing effectiveness of interventions ('to what extent does it work?'). There is another useful byproduct of understanding the different strengths and weaknesses of the different evidence types. The discerning reader will also have noticed that the different designs yield different types of knowledge for decision-makers. So depending on the question to be addressed, a particular design will be more appropriate (accepting that the method has greater potential for error on the cause and effect front the lower it is in the hierarchy). For example, to examine the prognosis for a health condition (the longer term outlook) a cohort study might be more useful, and for assessing causation the cohort and case-control studies might be the better designs.

The ABCD type grid helps us to know the strengths and limitations of the evidence, alerts us to taking extra caution when using different evidence types to inform decisions, and highlights when further research is needed in the area.

Things that evidence-users need to be able to do

As a decision-maker or other user of evidence, you will need to be able to:

- make sense of a report in front of you;
- understand what you are asking for and its limitations when asking someone else to look at the evidence base for you;
- be able to critically appraise a primary study even if you do not do this on a day-to-day basis.

You will now have the tools to be able to work out what you are dealing with and will be more aware of the strengths and limitations of your request if ever asking for the evidence base for a particular intervention or initiative. To feel even more confident you need to be able to critically appraise a primary study even if you do not do this on a daily basis.

Critical appraisal

Assessment of the methodological quality of primary studies is known as critical appraisal and there is an extensive literature relating to critical appraisal and its role in supporting evidence-based practice.[21,22,23] All evidence-users, whether decision-makers or not, should develop these basic skills as part of their professional development if their background has not covered this already. Whatever your starting point you can build on these skills as you practise them.

Here are some key questions as a starting point. They apply to all study types.

- Is the study question an important one for health and healthcare?
- Is the question described purposefully for use (in a meaningful way for 'practitioners' in their area of work)?
- Does the context apply to my population?
- Are the methods used sensible?
- Are potential biases and confounders discussed? (Some characteristics of studies can increase the certainty of the findings and some can reduce it).[5]
- Are the conclusions sensible?

- To what extent is there a need to improve on current treatments and activities? Or what risks will be reduced?
- How should the findings shape or change our decision-making, or not?
- Who wrote it? Note any potential incentives not to write in the public interest.
- And after you have read it, who should I be sharing this with who might not have seen it?

These questions and the basic hierarchy in Table 6.1 should get you started with more evidence aware decision-making.

Have an evidence gathering system

If you are in any way a decision-maker (of services or decisions in the clinical setting), have a workable system for accessing evidence when you need it and have a system for members of your team also. For example, you may be using an internet-based search facility to access reports and studies. Seek advice from your local health service librarian to advise on this for initial access. Training and ongoing support in evidence retrieval and appraisal should be part of routine staff development for those whose work is related to the commissioning of services. Box 6.1 is a suggested approach to gathering the evidence available on your subject of interest.

Use an evidence hierarchy as an everyday tool

As a decision-maker, many of the papers that come across your desk will not be presented in a research paper fashion. Do not be deterred by this. The principles of the evidence hierarchy will still be useful to help you make sense of the evidence in front of you for taking a particular course of action. There may be key words (e.g. meta-analysis, or controlled trial, or consensus statement) that provide clues as to the highest grade of evidence the conclusions are based on. For example, a briefing paper on the benefits of brisk walking might not be presented in an obvious study format but within the narrative it might clearly reference that the learning is from a meta-analysis which indicates the association of walking on cardiovascular fitness.[28]

> ## Box 6.1 **For gathering evidence, you could start with this . . .**
>
> (1) Use available guidelines from organizations that use explicit methods in their literature appraisal. For example, the National Institute for Health and Care Excellence (NICE),[25] Scottish Intercollegiate Guidelines Network,[24] and professional bodies (such as the Royal College of Obstetricians and Gynaecologists, Royal College of Physicians).
> (2) Search for systematic reviews using the research databases e.g. Cochrane database,[26] 'PubMed'[27] search facilities, or equivalent, to make sure (1) is up-to-date.
> (3) If no systematic reviews are found on your topic, look for primary research via your research database resources.
> (4) If no research information is available, use a general search or discuss with a local expert but be alert to increasing potentials for bias at this level, even if unintentional.
>
> Use your evidence hierarchy alertness throughout when exploring these.

Other research evidence

You will now be familiar with a range of studies from the evidence hierarchy that are used to answer questions of cause and effect, effectiveness of interventions, and how common things are. Two more types of research evidence that can also provide important information for decision-making and commissioning of services need to be mentioned. These are economic studies and qualitative studies. These provide complementary knowledge to that gathered from looking at cause and effect and intervention studies. Essentially, economic studies are useful to commissioners as they address questions of cost and use of resources. A well designed RCT might include this information or the study might be an economic evaluation in its own right. Different types of economic evaluation are described in Chapter 8 ('Purposeful Use of Health Intelligence'). Qualitative studies explore behaviours, understanding, and beliefs; these types of learning can add richness to the knowledge gathering about effectiveness of interventions.

Qualitative research

In decision-making you will also come across and use evidence from qualitative research. The term derives from a distinction between quantitative (numerical based) and qualitative (thematic and non-numerical sense-making) methods and the distinction is probably overemphasized. In reality the two are complementary and are different means of gathering information about the problem. As a commissioner or decision-maker surveying the best available evidence to help you understand what is happening and what you can practically achieve for your population, you will need to draw on knowledge collection methods deemed both qualitative and quantitative. For example, you may be concerned about the number of women who are smokers at the time of delivering their baby. You may have a prevalence estimate of say 12% for your population of delivering mothers from a quantitative data collecting method. But, what stopped the women giving up smoking during their pregnancy? This latter question would be better explored using a qualitative method to generate a richer understanding of the issues than a quantitative approach alone allows.

Qualitative methods include group observation (as a participant or as an observer), analysis of documents, focus groups, and in-depth interviewing. The process can be iterative as new learning refines the ongoing research method. Analysis of the narrative data is largely thematic (content analysis). To improve the validity of the findings, the results from several methods looking at the same topic may be taken into account; this type of sense-making is known as 'triangulation'.[29] There are several types of triangulation but overall it can be thought of as a strategy to test validity through the convergence of information from different sources. Findings can also be analysed by more than one researcher to improve validity.

Qualitative knowledge can be used to explore themes which can later be tested further by quantitative methods. Remember that the basic evidence hierarchy is primarily to discern the robustness of methods used to assess cause and effect. If one wonders where qualitative methods might lie on such an evidence hierarchy, it is important to note that qualitative studies are not usually designed to measure cause and effect, so using a classic evidence hierarchy of cause and effect with qualitative studies would be a clumsy application of it. More conducive ways to assess the robustness of contributions from qualitative studies include using explicit criteria to look at how well a purported study design has been conducted and analysed and can be useful in that respect, though clearly this approach is not based on a hierarchy of one qualitative method over another as such.[30] An assessment of the evidence produced can also be made using GRADE principles.[7] Knowledge from qualitative studies is probably better understood as a sphere of hypothesis generating and contextual knowledge which can help decision-makers. As such this sphere of enquiry would overlap with the classic evidence hierarchy more at the hypothesis-generating end rather than at the intervention end. Qualitative findings help to complete our understanding of real-life problems.

Use your skills

You will now be familiar with the main research-based evidence types that assess effectiveness of interventions and cause and effect. You will also be aware of the complementary contextual knowledge available from qualitative techniques. Basic critical appraisal considerations apply to all studies. All are relevant to decision-making for population health gain.

Be confident about what you can do and build on it.

Try it. You might even enjoy it!

Reflection

Think about a decision that you were part of in the last two weeks. Was the level of evidence that the decision was based on clear?

Think about an initiative in the local or national news that has caught your attention recently. What was the highest level of evidence that was based on?

'Quantitative methods are interested in learning about the certainties of the situation. Qualitative studies are interested in learning from the uncertainties of the situation.' To what extent do you agree with this statement?

References

1. Canadian Task Force on the Periodic Health Examination. The periodic health examination. *Can Med Assoc J* 1979;121(9):1193–1254.
2. Harbour R, Miller J. A new system for grading recommendations in evidence based guidelines. *BMJ* 2001;323:334–336.
3. Cochrane Consumer Network. Levels of evidence. Available at: https://consumers.cochrane.org/levels-evidence
4. Guyatt GH, Oxman AD, Vist GE et al. GRADE: an emerging consensus on rating quality of evidence and strength of recommendations. *BMJ* 2008;336:924.
5. Siemieniuk R, Guyatt G. What is GRADE. *BMJ Best Practice.* Available at: https://bestpractice.bmj.com/info/toolkit/learn-ebm/what-is-grade/
6. SIGN. Policy statement on the grading of recommendations in SIGN guidelines. Available at: https://www.sign.ac.uk/assets/sign_grading.pdf
7. NICE. Developing NICE guidelines: the manual process and methods PMG20, updated October 2018. Available at: https://www.nice.org.uk/process/pmg20/chapter/reviewing-research-evidence#assessing-quality-of-evidence-critical-appraisal-analysis-and-certainty-in-the-findings
8. Langlois EV, Daniels K, Akl EA. Evidence synthesis for health policy and systems. A methods guide. WHO, 2018.
9. Higgins JPT, Green S (eds). *Cochrane Handbook for Systematic Reviews of Interventions,* version 5.1.0, updated March 2011. The Cochrane Collaboration, 2011. Available at: http://www.handbook.cochrane.org
10. ISIS-2 (Second International Study of Infarct Survival) Collaborative Group. A randomised trial of streptokinase, oral aspirin, both, or neither among 17,187 cases of suspected myocardial infarction. *Lancet* 1988;332(8607):349–360.
11. ISIS-3 (Third International Study of Infarct Survival) Collaborative Group. A randomised comparison of streptokinase vs tissue plasminogen activator vs anistreplase and of aspirin plus heparin vs aspirin alone among 41,299 cases of suspected acute myocardial infarction. *Lancet* 1992;339(8796):753–770.
12. ISIS-4 (Fourth International Study of Infarct Survival) Collaborative Group. A randomised factorial trial assessing early oral captopril, oral mononitrate, and intravenous magnesium sulphate in 58,050 patients with suspected acute myocardial infarction. *Lancet* 1995;345(8951):669–682.
13. ISIS-1 (First International Study of Infarct Survival) Collaborative Group. A randomised trial of intravenous atenolol among 16,027 cases of suspected acute myocardial infarction. *Lancet* 1986;328(8498):57–66.
14. Marmot MG, Rose G, Shipley M, Hamilton PJS. Employment grade and coronary heart disease in British civil servants. *J Epidemiol Community Health* 1978;32:244–249.
15. Marmot MG, Stansfield S, Patel C et al. Health inequalities among British civil servants: the Whitehall II study. *Lancet* 1991;337(8754):1387–1393.
16. Doll R, Bradford Hill A. Smoking and carcinoma of the lung: preliminary report. *Br Med J* 1950; 2(4682):739–748.

17. Doll R, Bradford Hill A. The mortality of doctors in relation to their smoking habits: a preliminary report. *Br Med J* 1954;228:1451–1455.
18. Doll R, Bradford Hill A. Lung cancer and other causes of death in relation to smoking. A second report on the mortality of British doctors. *Br Med J* 1956;2(5001):1071–1081.
19. Gottlieb MS, Schanker HM, Fan PT et al. Pneumocystis pneumonia – Los Angeles. *MMWR* 1981;30(21):1–3.
20. Hymes KB, Cheung T, Greene JB et al. Kaposi's sarcoma in homosexual men – a report of eight cases. *Lancet* 1981;2(8247):598–600.
21. Sackett DL, Richardson WS, Rosenberg WMC, Haynes RB. *Evidence based medicine: how to practice and teach EBM.* Churchill-Livingstone, 1996.
22. Crombie IM. *The Pocket Guide to Critical Appraisal.* BMJ Publishing Group, 1996.
23. Greenhalgh T. How to read a paper: assessing the methodological quality of published papers. *BMJ* 1997;315:305.
24. Scottish Intercollegiate Guidelines Network. Available at: https://www.sign.ac.uk/
25. NICE. Available at: https://www.nice.org.uk/
26. Cochrane Library. Available at: https://www.cochranelibrary.com/
27. US National Library of Medicine. Available at: https://www.ncbi.nlm.nih.gov/pubmed
28. Public Health England. 10 minutes brisk walking each day in mid-life for health benefits and towards achieving physical activity recommendations. Evidence summary. Gateway number 2017294. August 2017.
29. Paton MQ. *Qualitative Research and Evaluation Methods.* 4th edition. SAGE publications, 2014.
30. Daly J, Willis K, Small R et al. A hierarchy of evidence for assessing qualitative health research. *J Clin Epidemiol* 2007;60(1):43–49.

7
Spectrum of Effective Preventive Opportunities

This vantage point is quite versatile and can be deployed in many of the situations and discussions you might come across in a commissioning role. It is probably the most subtly powerful of the vantage points for commissioners, being of use in matters of process and at a strategic level. Whilst its individual components may seem familiar, it is actually a multi-layered concept with wider practical applications than initially meets the eye. Any apparent simplicity does not diminish its potential in enabling more strategic thinking in whole system and service planning. The principles can be applied to a wide range of issues from the relatively straightforward to more complex scenarios.

Spotting effective preventive opportunities in any condition is crucial for improving healthcare effectiveness. These opportunities are important because they are opportunities to reduce the risk of poorer health outcomes and in turn, the need for health and care services further down the line (rather like turning down the flow of water from a tap). Whilst key messages in this chapter would be equally applicable to practice at the individual level, the focus of the chapter will be at the population level, which is of course the focus of this book.

Main points to be familiar with . . .

- What is an effective preventive opportunity.
- Using a 'Spectrum of Preventive Opportunities' as a strategic way of thinking about this for your practice.

Effective preventive opportunities

These are opportunities in the natural history of a condition or in a service care pathway, in which there is a feasible intervention to reduce the

Commissioning and a Population Approach to Health Services Decision-Making. Julie Sin, Oxford University Press (2020). © Oxford University Press. DOI: 10.1093/oso/9780198840732.001.0001

risk of ill-health or reduce the need for health services at a later point in time.

The emphasis on *'effective'* refers to using an evidence-based approach to identify interventions that work in real-life settings and are acceptable to the population. The emphasis on *'preventive'* refers to an intervention's impact on reducing future burden of disease in the population. This means that prevention applies not only to the prevention of the onset of a condition but also includes all actions and treatments that diminish recurrences or further disability. That is, the notion of prevention does not stop once a condition has been identified; there are preventive roles from there on as well.

Effective preventive opportunities are critical junctures in improving health service effectiveness. By considering where these opportunities lie along a care-pathway it helps the commissioning process to gain a system-wide view of effective options before embarking on a particular course of action. The approach can be used with any health condition, health status, or patient cohort e.g. coronary heart disease, frailty, or 0–5 year olds respectively. This approach can also help when working with partner agencies across the whole health and social care system.

Within this mix, we must also acknowledge that we do not yet have sufficient knowledge about the early development of all conditions to be able to prevent the onset of every condition that is seen by health services, and for the care of individuals with such conditions it is important that we continue to provide effective treatment and ongoing care until earlier opportunities to intervene become apparent. There are many examples of such conditions where preventing onset remains elusive at this juncture, but there are opportunities to slow down or reduce further morbidity and disability. Examples include autoimmune diseases such as rheumatoid arthritis, many neurodegenerative diseases such as Parkinson's disease, and rarer cancers to name but a few.

Preventive opportunities can therefore be thought of on a spectrum and a 'spectrum of preventive opportunities' is a strategic way of thinking about this.

A 'spectrum of preventive opportunities'

Take a moment to consider Figure 7.1. The model represents a whole care pathway approach to identifying preventive opportunities for any condition or health problem. The model is illustrative to help discern the preventive opportunities in a population system within a range of health and care services. The column headings are a blend of the natural history of the

A pathway model to understand preventive opportunities for health gain

Model can be used to map and identify effective opportunities for health gain for any condition/condition group. Opportunities will lie at different points of the spectrum for different conditions and depends on the extent that the main modifiable factors are understood and effective interventions are available

Wider determinants of health	Life-style risk factors	Primary care opportunities	Secondary and tertiary care opportunities	Rehabilitation and rest of life care
Health impacts of social, economic, and environmental factors.	Modifiable behavioural risk factors.	A setting for managing presenting conditions and ongoing care. Can include primary*, secondary** and tertiary*** prevention opportunities.	A setting for managing presenting conditions and can include primary*, secondary** and tertiary*** prevention opportunities.	Prevention of further disability. A emphasis on quality of life, care and dignity. Mainly tertiary prevention
e.g. housing, poverty, worklessness, transport, social isolation, employment, education, early years environment.	e.g. smoking, alcohol, sedentary lifestyles, diet, drug misuse.	e.g. all earlier opportunities plus: Action on modifiable metabolic risk factors such as high blood pressure, diabetes. Population screening programmes	e.g. all earlier opportunities plus: A focus on effective specialist treatments and advice to reduce illness recurrence and severity	

Key: *   Primary prevention: relates to preventing the onset of a disease.
  **   Secondary prevention: relates to reducing the impact of a disease that has already occurred by halting its progress or by preventing recurrence. Many population screening programmes are examples of this.
  *** Tertiary prevention: relates to softening the impact of an ongoing condition to improve function and quality of life.

Figure 7.1   Spectrum of Preventive Opportunities: A pathway model to understand opportunities for health gain.

Copyright © Julie Sin 2018.

condition and service pathway response components to help illustrate the points at which one might locate these opportunities. It can be applied to any health problem or condition. On the left-hand-side of the spectrum are upstream pre-illness junctures where opportunities may exist and this part of the spectrum also acknowledges the health impacts of wider determinants. Though this may seem broad, it should not be dismissed by health services. Much public sector multiagency work needs to recognize the modifiable parts of this arena locally in their joint approach to working on their service-user pathways. Towards the right, the setting for opportunities becomes increasingly health-service based. For simplicity, health service opportunities have been described as based in primary care (general practice and community settings) and secondary care (hospital settings). Rehabilitation and rest of life care are represented on the far right, relating to situations where the underlying disease process cannot be altered but its impact may still be modified and managed. In real-life, preventive measures can be delivered in more than one care setting and the column headings may blur with one another, but the essence of the spectrum to understand and explore opportunities remains useful (and it is preferable to have potential overlaps in the case of this model than to miss a stage to locate the opportunities).

All effective measures that improve health outcomes can be considered within this model regardless of which column they may be conventionally associated with. It becomes intuitive when using this model to consider all healthcare interventions because even specialized treatments and procedures are in fact attempts to reduce the ongoing burden of disease and to reduce future health needs. Implicitly there is also an emphasis to identify the earliest effective preventive opportunity for consideration in each pathway as that may give rise to the largest health gains in a population.

Building a big picture of preventive opportunities for your topic

You can use this model with any condition. You may wish to try it as a multidisciplinary group, for example as a commissioning team or a clinical network, or by yourself. Identify the main known modifiable risk factors for your condition of interest. Then consider the effective opportunities to deal with the condition as a whole using the pathway columns as a guide. You do not have to start at any particular column but try to consider them all. There may be a relevant effective preventive opportunity (EPO) in several columns or just one or two, depending on the topic.

A worked example is shown in Box 7.1 for lung cancer. For orientation, you may wish to initially note why the condition (or outcome of interest) is an important one to consider, for example whether it is a cause of significant morbidity or premature mortality in the population, or a national priority. After noting the main modifiable risk factors, the columns in Figure 7.1 have been used to identify effective actions that could be taken to reduce the impact of lung cancer in the population.

Key effective preventive opportunities may be at different points of the spectrum for different conditions. For example, cervical cancer is another largely preventable cancer of which the understanding of its origins has developed substantially over the past 30 years. The main carcinogen (cancer causing agent) is a sexually transmittable infection, namely certain subtypes of the human papilloma virus (HPV). The main effective preventive opportunity is thus vaccination against those subtypes of HPV virus that are associated with the majority of cervical cancers in the population. For

Box 7.1 **Preventive opportunities example—Lung Cancer**

Impact description: Cancers are a main cause of premature deaths (deaths under 75 years of age) in the population[1] with lung cancers being one of the commonest cancers in men and women.[2] Effective earlier opportunities are important as most lung cancers present late to services when there is poor one-year survival.

Main modifiable risk factors: Tobacco smoking mainly, and to a far lesser population extent, radon gas and asbestos exposure. (Radon gas is present naturally from the normal decay of small quantities of radioactive substances in rocks and soils. It is present in small quantities in almost all air but inadequate ventilated conditions such as underground mines means it can be present in concentrations that can increase the risk of lung cancer. Asbestos is a risk factor for pleural mesothelioma, a particular type of lung cancer of the lining of the lung. Main risk factor is occupational exposure to asbestos through its manufacture or its use in the construction industry.[3])

Preventive opportunities

Wider determinants and lifestyle	Primary care and community setting opportunities	Secondary care, specialized services, rest-of-life care
Tobacco control policies e.g. tobacco duty, advertising, and sales controls (national and local opportunities).	Smoking cessation services.	Hospital no-smoking policies.
	Earlier presentation to services for prompt identification.	Prompt diagnosis.
Lifestyle changes ~with regard to tobacco smoking.	Prompt referral and treatment as appropriate.	Treatment modalities: chemotherapy, radiotherapy, and surgery as appropriate.
Health and safety legislation to reduce risk of occupational risks of radon and asbestos exposure.	[No effective screening programme opportunity at this point in time.]	Palliative care.

Summary: Best current prospect of reducing lung cancers in the population is to tackle the main modifiable risk factor which is tobacco smoking. A much smaller number of cases of lung cancer are also radon or asbestos related. Once cancer has developed, earlier presentation to services is associated with improved one-year survival. As with all pathways, remember to review as evidence evolves.

example in the UK there is a vaccination (immunization) programme offered to young people of secondary school age (first dose 12–13 years).[4] In addition to immunization, there is also a national cervical cancer screening programme, as not all such cancers will be prevented by immunization and there are many women in older cohorts who may already have been exposed to HPV subtypes of concern before the vaccination programme began. A preventive opportunities look at cervical cancer would therefore identify vaccination against HPV and cervical screening programme as the earliest preventive opportunities, with of course prompt diagnosis and treatment being part of the population spectrum of care to be in place as well.

For some cancers of course, there is no clear modifiable risk factor to prevent its onset in susceptible individuals, and neither is there an effective population screening programme to detect it at an early stage. Such examples include lymphoma, pancreatic, and neurological cancers. Prompt identification and ongoing care will remain the mainstay of provision for these patients and the main means of reducing premature mortality and morbidity from these conditions in the population until more is known. This is the same for many non-cancer conditions also, where there is as yet no clear specific risk factor that can be reduced to prevent its onset. Boxes 7.2 and 7.3 are examples of using the spectrum model to identify effective preventive opportunities where there is no early single risk factor that can be modified. The first relates to diabetes type 1 which is a condition that can affect many organ systems of the body if not managed. The other is osteoarthritis, a common cause of joint pain and reduced mobility in the older population.[5]

You will now have a flavour of how the spectrum can be used to gain a big picture of the opportunities to tackle your condition of interest. Try it. It does not matter if you do not have all the knowledge at your fingertips, it is the structured approach that helps. Use the skills of your team or

Box 7.2 **Preventive opportunities example—Diabetes type 1**

Impact description: A long-term health condition due to insufficient production of insulin by the pancreas so the body cannot finely tune blood sugar levels. It affects many aspects of a patient's life. Treatment and prevention of diabetic complications is lifelong. Untreated high levels of blood sugar leads to diabetic crises (ketoacidosis) and longer term vascular complications can affect many organs (heart and circulatory system, eyes, feet, peripheral nerves).

Main modifiable risk factors: Largely unknown. Some familial predisposition.

Preventive opportunities[6,7]

Wider determinants and lifestyle	Primary care and community setting opportunities	Secondary care, specialized services, rest-of-life care
Behavioural lifestyle changes to reduce the cumulative risks for diabetic complications (tobacco use, diet, physical exercise).	Insulin therapy, structured education, self-care, and primary care management of blood sugar levels and appropriate equipment to assist. Reduce modifiable metabolic risk factors: raised blood pressure, cholesterol. Prevention and management of complications of diabetes, including care to reduce risk of eye, foot, kidney, and circulatory disease.	Diabetologist review. Transition from paediatric to adult care. Obstetrician review for maternity care in diabetic patients. Audit and evaluate quality of care for improvements.

Summary: Cannot prevent onset in those susceptible but can manage the condition. Best current prospect of reducing impact of type 1 diabetes in the population is to support patients to manage their day-to-day care of blood sugar levels and insulin administration to reduce risk of hypoglycaemic episodes (low blood sugar due to more insulin administered than needed). Long-term management of the condition is very important to reduce the risk of diabetic complications to other organ systems. As with all pathways, remember to review as evidence evolves.

Box 7.3 Preventive opportunities example—Osteoarthritis

Impact description:[5,8] Osteoarthritis (OA) is the most common form of arthritis and one of the leading causes of pain and disability worldwide.[5] A degenerative condition, it involves structural changes of the affected joint causing pain and functional disability. Often more than one joint is involved. The main goal of treatment is to relieve joint pain and improve everyday physical function. It is a common underlying reason for hip and knee joint replacements. Prevalence of hip osteoarthritis and knee osteoarthritis in the UK is estimated to be 10.9% and 18.2% respectively, of people aged 45 years and over.[9]

Main modifiable risk factors: Upstream prevention of OA remains challenging. Mechanical factors such as joint injury (including that as a result of other joint disease) and malalignment appears to increase the risk of OA. Obesity can accelerate worsening of OA.[10]

Preventive opportunities:[8,11–14]

Wider determinants and lifestyle	Primary care and community setting opportunities	Secondary care, specialized services, rest-of-life care
No clear modifiable single factor, but physical activity and reduction in obesity would help to maintain muscle strength, mobility and fitness in the population.	Patient information. Exercise and physiotherapy. Analgesia. Weight management (if needed). Intra-articular injections for short-term symptom relief. Footwear, assistive devices (e.g. walking aids, tap turners). Referral for consideration of joint surgery.	Joint surgery for end-stage disease. Other orthopaedic procedures. Post-operative mobilization.

Summary: Cannot prevent onset in those susceptible but can manage the condition. Best current prospect of reducing impact of OA in the population is pain management, exercise as symptoms allow to maintain muscle strength, joint mobility, and balance. Conservative treatment is the mainstay of care. Joint replacement may be possible in appropriate cases. Review as evidence evolves.

multidisciplinary network as needed. With a multidisciplinary team it is usually quite intuitive and a range of insights can be offered. For completeness and if needed, Boxes 7.4 and 7.5 might help as prompts about types of risk factors and interventions.

Box 7.4 **Population health 'sieve'**

Risk factor processes in the population:

- Social, economic, and environmental factors (wider determinants of health);
- Genetics and age;
- Lifestyle—Addictive substances (tobacco, alcohol, illicit drugs);
- Lifestyle—Nutritional health and physical activity (overweight and obesity, low fruit and vegetable intake, physical inactivity, malnutrition);
- Metabolic risk factors (high blood pressure, high blood glucose, high LDL cholesterol);
- Pathogens (infectious organisms);
- Degenerative (the result of a continuous process of deterioration in cells and tissues over time);
- Access to effective healthcare, social care, and wider support in the community;
- Iatrogenic (associated with treatment and care) e.g. pressure ulcers, healthcare associated infections;
- Idiopathic (unexplained).

Box 7.5 Intervention type

People-facing:

- Advice and support at population level (e.g. awareness raising);
- Drugs;
- Devices;
- Procedures (can be minor or major), including screening procedures;
- Individual care and support;
- Physical therapies;
- 'Talking therapies' (e.g. cognitive behavioural therapy, family therapy);
- Multifaceted (combination of the above).

System-facing:
Related to organization of care.

- Effectiveness of services;
- Clinical pathways;
- Information technology;
- Professionals providing the care.

Uses of the model

The model can be used as a communication and reference tool to support:

- strategic commissioning. It can be applied at a local level or any larger footprint. For example, CCG, clinical network, and integrated working footprints between health and social care;
- resource allocation within pathways;
- defining care pathway junctures where effectiveness of services should be monitored and evaluated;
- multidisciplinary communications within and across organizations about improving health outcomes;

- identifying priorities for future research, for example, gaps in knowledge about causation (aetiology) and effectiveness of different types of intervention and care.

Types of predisposing and causal risk factors

Clinicians may be familiar with using a 'surgical sieve' to think about the root causal processes of medical and surgical conditions to help guide appropriate medical and surgical management. A similar approach can be used at the population level as a guide to thinking about where preventive opportunities might lie in a health system. Box 7.4 is a summary of such factors. Clearly some factors are potentially modifiable, others such as genetics are not.

The causation of a health condition can be an interplay of more than one factor (multifactorial). For example there may be a genetic predisposition and then an environmental trigger factor that may increase the risk of the disease occurring. Diseases can also be idiopathic. That is, as far as we can discern at this point in time the disease has occurred spontaneously, with no identifiable causal factors. Nevertheless the list can be a useful prompt to structure thinking about causal risk factors.

The directness of impact

Risk factors can have *direct proximal effects* on health (e.g. hypertension, adverse lipid ratios, infectious agent, smoking, alcohol, obesity, physical inactivity), or more *distal effects* (education, income, 'wider determinants'). In general, the more distal the effect the greater the likelihood that agencies other than health and care services may have a more direct role in influencing the effect. The more direct the effect the more likely it is to be addressed via health services. This is useful when considering which agencies and assets in the system could influence this. This connects risk factor understanding with how different agencies might have the best opportunity to make a difference or collaborate to make a difference.

A risk factor can of course be related to more than one health condition. For example, with non-communicable diseases (such as cardiovascular disease, chronic respiratory disease, cancers, and diabetes), four particular behaviours (tobacco use, physical inactivity, unhealthy diets, and harmful use of alcohol) and air pollution are implicated in leading to key physiological changes in the body (high blood pressure, obesity/overweight, raised blood glucose, and raised blood cholesterol) which increases the risk for disease development.[15]

Types of health system interventions

Box 7.5 can be used to consider the types of intervention and care processes that may be effective in the situation of interest.

Using a spectrum approach to examine system level topics

Earlier examples have looked at specific conditions. The following examples illustrate how the approach can also be applied to gather insights about a whole-system pathway (Box 7.6), or a specific group of patients (Box 7.7). In these examples it may make sense to merge some of the original columns together, as many of the opportunities are system facing or have particular interdependencies with other system contributions.

Nomenclature: Stages of prevention

The terms primary, secondary, and tertiary prevention are sometimes used to categorize preventive efforts. For interest and to avoid confusion they are worth a further note here for orientation.

Primary prevention refers to actions that aim to prevent the onset of a health condition. For example, smoking cessation to reduce the risk of cardiovascular disease and cancers, immunizations against childhood infections, and seat-belt legislation to reduce injury from road traffic accidents. Secondary prevention refers to actions, after the onset of disease, to prevent the disease progressing further or recurring. Examples are the early detection of breast cancer through mammography screening, or medication after a heart attack or stroke to reduce the risk of another event. Tertiary prevention refers to reducing disability from the condition when the course of the disease process cannot be altered. Effectiveness at this point tends to focus on quality of life.

Box 7.6 Example—'Winter Pressures'

Impact description: This refers to the increased demands on health and social care services over the winter season (November to March), but can be present at any time of year. The term can be used narrowly to refer to how hospitals cope with the challenges of maintaining regular service over the winter period, although there may be similar capacity challenges in other parts of the health and care delivery system. It is best considered as a whole health and care system issue. It results from the combined effects of seasonal increase in morbidity[16] and structural problems in the healthcare system (how the system is set up and its processes). A surge in demand of patients with severe and complex needs can significantly affect accident and emergency departments and in turn, the access to beds of the rest of the hospital as a whole.

Vulnerable groups: older people, particularly over 75 years who are frail and socially isolated, the very young, chronically ill, and those with reduced ability to self-care.[17]

Main risk factors:

Factors increasing illness in individuals: Cold weather, circulating influenza and influenza-like illnesses affecting already vulnerable people. Also temporal trends in population age distribution leading to greater numbers of people with multiple morbidities and needs of greater complexity.

Structural issues in healthcare: Factors that limit resilience in the system to cope with increased demand for hospital care. These include when:

- bed occupancy rates are high as a norm, there is reduced flexibility to respond to additional pressures (e.g. occupancy rates over 93% in 2016/17 and 2017/18).[18] (As more elective surgery over the years has been performed as day cases, the number of inpatient beds has reduced);
- there are delays in being able to arrange community nursing and/ or social care for hospital patients who are otherwise medically fit for discharge which can reduce *'flow'* of patients through hospital as well as being a suboptimal setting for patients;
- there are capacity issues with *interdependent services* e.g. community nursing, social care, primary care.

Most structural issues are modifiable in principle.

Preventive opportunities[17,19]

Wider determinants, lifestyle and general community opportunities (individual and system-facing approaches)	Primary care, other community settings, hospital care, and rest-of-life opportunities (individual and system-facing approaches)
• Warmth and heating (home insulation, draught-proofing, clothing).	• Opportunistic engagement about cold weather advice for those in contact with services ('making every contact count' approach).
• Nutrition (hot food and drinks) and mobility.	• 'Flu (influenza) vaccinations for groups at higher risk of severe disease and frontline health and care workers.
• Measures to reduce fuel poverty.	• Advice about having sufficient medicines at home for chronic conditions and asymptomatic relief of minor ailments.
• Local plans to ensure local people are contacted.	• Review capacity and access to community health and social care.
• Checking on those at risk, living alone.	• Coordination among local health and care system providers to consider the increases in demand from the classically vulnerable and the 'non-vulnerable' groups.
• Self-care advice.	• Primary care, hospital staff, and other recruitment issues to be attended to before season starts, as much as possible.
• Awareness raising about pharmacy-based minor ailments services.	• Active optimization of care of frail patients to start before hospital discharge (e.g. medicines review, physiotherapy assessment so eventual discharge is not delayed).
	• Balance between number of beds (and staff) needed for a high bed occupancy rate and that needed for optimal throughput in winter
	• Protocols for improved patient flow and safety[20] (e.g. senior review, estimated discharge date, discharge earlier in the day, active review of patients staying more than seven days).

Summary: Best prospect of managing demand is a system-wide population approach across health and social care both in reducing risks from individual factors, and increasing system resilience. Review as evidence evolves for these pathways.

Box 7.7 Example—Severe Mental Illness (SMI)

Impact description: The term is usually used to refer to psychotic disorders, often defined by their length of duration and the disability they produce.[21] Psychoses are a cluster of disorders with variable expression in which a person's perceptions, thoughts, mood, and behaviour are significantly altered. Typically these conditions have far-reaching consequences for multiple domains of the lives of those who experience them. The NHS Quality and Outcomes Framework (QOF) indicator for severe mental illness encompasses schizophrenia, bipolar disorder, other psychoses, and other patients receiving lithium.[22] Schizophrenia is the most frequently encountered psychotic illness. Schizophrenia has a point prevalence averaging around 0.45% and a lifetime expectancy of 0.7%, although there is considerable variation in different areas and a higher risk in urban environments.[23] Prevalence with the QOF definition was 0.9% in 2016–17.[22]

Main risk factors: Aetiology (causal processes) is poorly understood. No single modifiable risk factor is known. There appears to be a complex interplay of environmental factors with genetic susceptibility. It is unclear how they fit together.[24,25]

Stressors include: parental antisocial behaviour and substance use, parental mental illness, child abuse, early substance misuse, deviant peer relationships, family disruption, low popularity among peers, and impoverished and socially disorganized neighbourhoods with high levels of crime. However, some people with SMI may have experienced none of these.

People with severe mental illness also have worse physical health outcomes, and premature mortality is much greater in people with SMI than in the general population. Much of this is due to increased risks for cardiovascular disease.[1,21]

Preventive opportunities to reduce the burden of illness of SMIs

Wider determinants, lifestyle, and general community opportunities (individual and system-facing opportunities).[26]	Primary care, other community settings, hospital care, and rest-of-life opportunities (individual and system-facing opportunities).
General strategies to improve population resilience. Improving nutrition, housing, and access to education; reducing economic insecurity; community networks, reducing harm from addictive substances. *Reducing impact of stressors:* Promoting a healthy start in life, reducing child neglect and abuse, coping with parental mental illness, enhancing resilience and reducing risk behaviour in schools, dealing with family disruption.	• Prompt referral for assessment of those suspected to have a SMI.[27,28,29] • Effective primary and secondary care interface to enable prompt referral.[27] • Specialist mental health teams in community and inpatient settings. • Antipsychotic medications (primary treatment for schizophrenia and other psychoses). • Psychosocial therapies e.g. cognitive behavioural therapy and family intervention. • Crisis resolution and home treatment teams. • Comprehensive physical assessment, including physical exercise and nutrition programme, and help to stop smoking. • Social support to improve ability to live independently. • Interventions to offer employment and vocational training. • Support for carers.

Summary: Whilst the aetiology of SMI is poorly understood, the mental, physical, and social consequences for affected individuals and carers can be severe and lifelong. The best current prospect of reducing the impact of SMIs in the population is a multifaceted approach of strategies to improve population resilience, and for prompt identification, referral, diagnosis, and ongoing management of affected individuals.

The terminology can sometimes be useful in practice, but beware; though the terms may be understood as described above, they can sometimes become mistakenly aligned with the terms 'primary care', 'secondary care', and 'tertiary care' during multi-professional discussions. The latter terms, of course, refer to settings in which healthcare can be accessed and are completely independent descriptive terms with no exclusive or direct alignment to the categorizations of primary, secondary, and tertiary prevention. (That is, primary prevention does not necessarily mean that the preventive activity is delivered from a primary care setting (though it could be), nor should activities termed secondary prevention infer that it is delivered from a secondary care setting, etc.)

If the terms primary, secondary, and tertiary prevention become more confusing as a communication tool than they are helpful, it is probably best to use something else in the situation. A focus on identifying 'effective preventive opportunities' for a population's health using a care pathway spectrum approach would be a more facilitative approach. The latter will intuitively capture all the 'stages of prevention' with tangible delivery points in a physical system, and may avoid any misconceptions that primary prevention is the sole territory of primary care, or secondary prevention is territory of secondary care, etc.

Another pitfall that sometimes scuppers system efforts to optimize effective preventive opportunities is that in everyday parlance the generic use of the word prevention might only be understood more narrowly as those aspects of prevention that are primary prevention. Whilst that might sometimes be sufficient for general usage it is insufficient for health service decision-makers who have responsibility for reducing the burden of disease in the population through opportunities across the whole health system. The spectrum helps planners of health and care to avoid this trap and allows consideration of all care pathway opportunities.

Underused opportunities

Remember that even when an effective preventive opportunity is clearly recognized it could still be under-deployed within the population. For example, the role of tobacco smoking and its links to cardiovascular disease, respiratory disease, and a range of cancers are well known but there are still opportunities to reduce this risk factor further to reduce longer term harm in the population, for example through ongoing reduction in population smoking prevalence rates, 'smoke free' hospitals, and reduction of smoking in pregnancy. Similarly, there remain gains to be made with respect to alcohol intake and physical inactivity in the population. Identification and control of hypertension, atrial fibrillation, and raised blood glucose in the population are further effective preventive measures that could be more widespread across the population.

Ready for action

You will now be familiar with the spectrum of preventive opportunities. It can be applied to any care pathway. The model can also be used to consider system level topics and groups of conditions. It helps to flush out potential 'people-facing' and 'system-facing' preventive opportunities for overall understanding of the topic. This context is relevant for decision-making for population health gain.

Reflection

Consider a health issue you are familiar with. To your knowledge, what are the main known modifiable causative factors, if any? Of those, for which ones are there known effective interventions that could make a difference to the outcome?

Effective preventive efforts to reduce risk of future adverse outcomes in the population have an effect. Although names cannot be put to all those that have benefited, we may be able to estimate the number of people who have benefited compared with if no action had been taken. These 'statistical beneficiaries' of averted adverse outcomes are real lives.

Do statistical beneficiaries feel as real as the more identifiable named beneficiaries of health service treatments and procedures in the population?

If one situation feels more real than the other, is that actually so? How might that affect health services decision-making?

References

1. Department of Health. Living well for longer: national support for local action to reduce premature avoidable mortality. Crown copyright, 2014.
2. Office for National Statistics. Cancer registration statistics, England: 2016. Updated June 2018. Available at: https://www.ons.gov.uk/peoplepopulationandcommunity/healthandsocialcare/conditionsanddiseases/bulletins/cancerregistrationstatisticsengland/final2016#breast-prostate-lung-and-colorectal-cancers-continue-to-be-the-most-common
3. Macmillan Cancer Support. Risk factors and causes of pleural mesothelioma. Available at: https://www.macmillan.org.uk/information-and-support/mesothelioma/pleural-mesothelioma/diagnosing/causes-and-risk-factors
4. NHS. HPV vaccine. 2017. Available at: https://www.nhs.uk/conditions/vaccinations/hpv-human-papillomavirus-vaccine/
5. Cross M, Smith F, Hoy D et al. The global burden of hip and knee osteoarthritis: estimates from the Global Burden of Disease 2010 study. *Ann Rheum Dis* 2014;73:1323–1330.
6. NICE. Type 1 diabetes in adults: diagnosis and management. NICE guideline [NG17], updated July 2016.
7. NICE. Diabetes (type 1 and type 2) in children and young people: diagnosis and management. NICE guideline [NG18], updated November 2016.
8. NICE. Osteoarthritis: care and management. Clinical guideline [CG177]. February 2014.
9. Public Health England. Musculoskeletal diseases profile. June 2018. Available at: https://fingertips.phe.org.uk/profile/msk
10. Neogi T, Zhang Y. Osteoarthritis Prevention. *Curr Opin Rheumatol* 2011 Mar;23(2): 185–191.
11. Uthman OA, van der Windt DA, Jordan J, Dziedzic KS, Healey EL, Peat GM et al. Exercise for lower limb osteoarthritis: systematic review incorporating trial sequential analysis and network meta-analysis. *BMJ* 2013;347:f5555.
12. Fransen M, McConnell S, Harmer AR, Van der Esch M, Simic M, Bennell KL. Exercise for osteoarthritis of the knee: a Cochrane systematic review. *Br J Sports Med* 2015; 49:1554–1557.
13. NICE. Total hip replacement and resurfacing arthroplasty for end-stage arthritis of the hip. Technology appraisal guidance [TA304]. February 2014.
14. NICE. Osteoarthritis. Quality standard [QS87]. June 2015.
15. WHO. Noncommunicable diseases, country profiles 2018.
16. NHS England and NHS Improvement. Quick guide: planning for increased seasonal demand in respiratory illness. 2017.
17. Public Health England and NHS England. The cold weather plan for England, protecting health and reducing harm from cold weather. Gateway numbers 2015382 and 04153. October 2015.
18. British Medical Association. NHS pressures, winter analysis. 2018.

19. Public Health England and NHS England. The cold weather plan for England, making the case: why long term strategic planning for cold weather is essential to health and well-being. Gateway numbers 2015382 and 04152. 2017.
20. NHS Improvement. The SAFER patient flow bundle. Available at: https://improvement.nhs.uk/documents/633/the-safer-patient-flow-bundle.pdf
21. Royal College of Psychiatrists. Working Group for Improving the Physical Health of People with SMI. Improving the physical health of adults with severe mental illness: essential actions (OP100). 2016.
22. NHS Employers. 2016/17 General Medical Services (GMS) contract Quality and Outcomes Framework (QOF), Guidance for GMS contract 2016/17. Gateway reference 05093. April 2016.
23. van Os J, Kenis G, Rutten BP. The environment and schizophrenia. *Nature* 2010; 468:203–212.
24. van Os J, Linscott RJ, Myin-Germeys I, Delespaul P, Krabbendam L. A systematic review and meta-analysis of the psychosis continuum: evidence for a psychosis proneness-persistence-impairment model of psychotic disorder. *Psychol Med* 2009;39:179–195.
25. Tandon R, Keshavan MS, Nasrallah HA. Schizophrenia, 'just the facts', what we know in 2008. 2. Epidemiology and etiology. *Schizophr Res* 2008;102:1–18.
26. WHO. Prevention of mental disorders: effective interventions and policy options. Summary report/ a report of the World Health Organization Dept. of Mental Health and Substance Abuse; in collaboration with the Prevention Research Centre of the Universities of Nijmegen and Maastricht. 2004.
27. NICE. Psychosis and schizophrenia in adults. Quality standard 80 [QS80]. February 2015.
28. NICE. Psychosis and schizophrenia in adults: prevention and management Clinical guideline [CG178]. Updated March 2014. Available at: http://www.nice.org.uk/guidance/CG178
29. NICE. Bipolar disorder: assessment and management. Clinical Guideline [CG185]. Updated April 2018. Available at: https://www.nice.org.uk/guidance/cg185

8
Purposeful Use
of Health Intelligence

There are much routine data available. Generation of new data is labour intensive and does not always answer the pertinent questions, so data and information need to be used purposefully. This chapter considers how commissioners can frame the questions they pose of health information sources, so that they gain more meaningful answers to help commission for health gain.

As a decision-maker you will need to make sense of situations. The purposeful use of health data and information is one aspect that will help you to do that. Chapter 6 has looked at evidence from the research literature that can inform commissioning. That is one type of tangible knowledge or intelligence for decision-making. The knowledge available from routine statistics and numerical datasets often described as health information is another source. This chapter focuses on the use of this routine statistical information for commissioning.

Health information, whether derived routinely from health service interactions or specifically collected, can be used to help the planning of services. Whilst there may be a whole behind-the-scenes supporting infrastructure to gather, organize, and quality assure this rich repository of health information,[1,2] the challenge remains for commissioners and decision-makers that any repository needs to be used in tangible ways for it to improve health and inequalities in the population.

Routinely available health information spans a myriad of population statistics, healthcare processes, and health condition pathways (for example information about liver disease, diabetes, or cancers). This breadth and volume available may initially seem impenetrable to the practitioner who wants to use it to guide their commissioning or to improve the quality of their local services. The emphasis of this chapter is concerned with making use of health information from a commissioning perspective.

Commissioning and a Population Approach to Health Services Decision-Making. Julie Sin, Oxford University Press (2020). © Oxford University Press. DOI: 10.1093/oso/9780198840732.001.0001

Main points to be familiar with ...

- Framing questions purposefully so that the information you gain can inform your commissioning or decision-making.
- The three main uses of health information in commissioning are closely related to the commissioning cycle activities.

Data, information, health intelligence

The following working definitions are used in this chapter:

> *Data* are facts or statistics collected together for reference or analysis.[3] If these health-related data are assembled meaningfully and presented in context, this produces *health information*. The application of the significance of the findings in real-life context, and putting this learning into decision-making that aims to improve health, is *health intelligence*.

Sometimes the terms health information and health intelligence are used interchangeably, although there is a subtle distinction between them in that health intelligence infers there is an intent to deploy the knowledge actively for a specific purpose to improve health and health services. Where there is a choice the term health intelligence will be used in the chapter as the generic term as that is the overall aim for the use of such data and information.

It is also useful to acknowledge that often the best available information falls short of all the information we would like and we are confronted with considering what is 'good enough' information to use. A pragmatic interpretation of good enough is that which is reasonable to assume is 'enough to set off in the right direction and/or incrementally improves our knowledge of the situation'. Combined with a continuous 'do, learn, and refine' approach where safe to so do, good enough is often sufficient to set off. It is a part of using our resources and efforts effectively.

Framing questions

A general note about the framing of questions is useful here. This is a relatively quick but important stage before interrogating any datasets or requesting health information. From experience it can often be given less thought than it deserves. In order to generate useful knowledge that will help to clarify a problem or help you make a decision, you should be asking purposeful questions. Although the focus of this chapter is concerned with questions with a health-information type answer, the basic principles about purposeful questions applies to all questions, whether they have a statistical or descriptive answer. You may already have your own methods of asking purposeful questions, but if not you could try considering the following checkpoints when forming your question.

Firstly, consider the framing of your question. Framing helps to focus on one issue among many others. It makes answering more manageable, helps to avoid getting 'bogged down' during the process, and makes the answer more useful. Of all the issues which could apply, which aspect or consequences are you focusing on? Is your question sufficiently framed if you were hearing it for the first time?

Secondly, consider clarity. Apart from steering you to the most appropriate information sources, thus saving you or someone else time, clarity will help you to recognize whether the question has been answered or not. Consider the purpose of the question, why you are asking, and what it is for. Consider whether any parts of the question are ambiguous and whether you have given sufficient definitions of what you need. For practical reasons and business expediency it is also helpful to let others know when the information is needed by and the format it is needed in.

Thirdly, and as importantly, consider the openness of your question. This refers to openness to hearing the answer whatever it might be, rather than having a preconceived range of acceptable answers.

Perhaps the best way to see the value of this is to consider an unfocused request such as, 'can you give me everything you have about older people?'. Whilst there may be many worthwhile issues to explore within the topic area of older people, as a question for interrogating health information resources, there is no clear health information question and there is insufficient framing. The questioner in this case would need to give the matter more thought before anyone can start looking at the data. The age group of older people is not defined, but even if that were known there is still no clear question. The pertinent question or questions might turn out to be about how many people live in the nursing homes in the area, or how many people are aged 65 and over, or how many people have a diagnosis of dementia, or about the old age dependency ratio, or about the number of carers, or how many people report having a limiting long-term illness, or living independently in single-person households, or one of many other possible questions. We will never know unless it is clarified and framed.

Try also to avoid questions like, 'what is the information to show we are a top performer for service X?'. This question lacks openness and does not consider the possibility that our service X might not perform well relative to other similar services. The question, 'how do the outcomes from our commissioned service X compare to outcomes of similar services in other similar population areas?' would have more openness. Openness allows you to see the issue from a perspective you might not have expected and might help you in managing situations in a more informed manner.

With these general principles in mind, we will now consider use of information in commissioning.

Use of health intelligence for commissioning: 'Just three things'

As part of an evidence-based approach, the effective use of health intelligence is a key ingredient in the pursuit of improving health and reducing health inequalities through commissioning.

Pragmatically, the use of health intelligence for commissioning tends to boil down to three main lines of enquiry (Box 8.1). You can use this to guide your initial framing of the question.

Box 8.1 **Three main uses of health intelligence for commissioning**

  (i) Intelligence to DEFINE and understand the problem(s).
 (ii) Intelligence to help PLAN and PRIORITIZE possible actions to address the problem(s).
(iii) Intelligence sources to MONITOR and EVALUATE outcomes and whether our efforts are effective.

This will make particular sense if you are familiar with the basic commissioning cycle (Chapter 4). From experience, this model can be used on a daily basis to help clarify the questions we should be seeking to answer with the available tools. It is a practical framework for thinking about the use of health information whether one has arrived at the question from a service development, public health, finance, research, or intelligence angle.

These considerations provide an initial framework to your information gathering, whether you are a requester of information or are about to interrogate a dataset yourself. For commissioning, your quest for new knowledge is then driven by your purposeful line of enquiry rather than by what happens to be in front of you. The array of indicators and products available then become tools at your disposal when you need them, rather than a large collection of information which is difficult to discern for relevance without this context. That is, your chosen line of questioning and the information you gain become intelligence for decision-making.

Benefits of the model

- To understand why requested health information is necessary (or not).
- To frame our questions more purposefully for commissioning.
- To understand what to do with the findings. This increases the likelihood that the findings will inform change that can improve health.

Example questions for health information

Box 8.2 contains example questions to help your thinking of questions for your own services and population of interest. Remember to use your multidisciplinary team to hone down your questions if needed. For ease of use, the examples have been grouped across the three areas of inquiry described in Box 8.1.

Getting started on the right foot with information

Remember datasets are simply sets of data. They do not necessarily align to a single question only. You frame your question then make use of the most appropriate information sources. The same item of information could be

Box 8.2 Examples of questions for health information

To define and understand the problem:

- How common is the issue in the population? (Look at incidence, prevalence or utilization rates as relevant, age–sex standardized if possible.)
- What has been the trend over the past ten years? (or other sensible time period).
- What is the prevalence of key risk factors?
- What is the premature mortality associated with this condition?
- What does the quality of life information with this condition show? (e.g. the 'disability-adjusted life years' impact of the condition).
- What proportion of those affected has sought the help of services?
- How does our population compare with comparator populations? (e.g. similar demographic populations or the country as a whole).
- What is the variation in access and outcomes of existing services (e.g. by geography, socioeconomic group, or other relevant local group), if any?

To plan and prioritize:
Many questions are possible depending on the nature of the intervention or service. Whether related to a community- or hospital-based service or a whole-population approach, the information sought usually relates to assessing the size and cost of a proposed solution to a problem and to gauge service usage:

- How many people would benefit from proposed intervention or service?
- Currently, how many community interactions/admissions to hospital/procedures take place per year for the condition in the population of interest?
- What are the routes of admission for this condition (electively or as an emergency)?

- What is the average 'length of stay' in hospital (or equivalent in the community) for the condition?
- What is the cost per admission/outpatient appointment/follow-up appointment/procedure?
- What is the rate and number of referrals from primary care for the service?
- What are the 'conversion rates' from referral to surgery/treatment (if appropriate)?
- How many avoidable delayed transfers of care occur per week?
- What is the uptake of services after invitation to attend (for example for screening programmes)?
- What does economic evaluation information say about the possible solutions in this topic?

To monitor and evaluate services:
Information is sought to inform what difference has been made, and whether services are delivering what has been agreed:

- How much has the service cost compared to contract expectations?
- What has been the effect on locally and nationally agreed outcome measures of the service?
- What is the available data on patient experience?
- What has been the effect on incidence/healthcare usage measures? (This might not demonstrate cause and effect but you would be interested to know if there has been any change).
- How many complaints and serious incidents (as defined by national guidance) have there been in the past year?
- What has been the effect on variations in access across geographical groups/socioeconomic groups?
- What has been the effect on uptake rates of services/ referrals from primary care/ length of stay in hospital?
- What is the premature mortality (deaths under 75 years) for the condition of interest?
- What has been the effect on rates of late-stage diagnosis and survival rates (if relevant)?

relevant for several aspects of commissioning enquiry depending on why it is needed. For example, information about incidence of a condition could be used to understand the nature of the issue at hand, or to plan a possible solution, or to assess whether an intervention has made a difference. This is why framing a question is important as the information can then be used purposefully when obtained.

In England there is much routine data available from accessible sources (Box 8.3). As data collation and analysis are very time consuming activities, the increased specialization of this function at a national and regional level to deliver quality-assured information for local geographical footprints can be very useful in practice.[2] The challenge for the commissioner is to use these sources discriminately to inform their commissioning activities.

For straightforward uses and orientation, the available sources, with the guidance of your local information analyst colleagues as needed, may be sufficient. Where the specific information you seek can only be collected by a bespoke interrogation and analysis, you may need to seek more in-depth advice from your information analyst resources. This may be a scarce resource so you will need to consider how the information you expect to gain will be used to inform the decision-making process, and whether the resources expended in producing this information are a good use of your or another's time.

Types of tangible knowledge needed for decision-making

At this juncture it is useful to remind ourselves that although health information can provide crucial knowledge to commissioning, it is not the only type of empirical knowledge you might need for decision-making. It is useful to remind ourselves that decision-making needs not only information from statistical data, but also knowledge of the evidence base of what works and of the local context.

So pragmatically, each of the following types of knowledge is important, but none is sufficient used alone for decision-making:

a. *Research evidence* of what works, to what extent it works, or does not work (see Chapter 6).
b. *Information from numerical-based data collection methods* (health information).

Box 8.3 **Routine sources of health information**

Much routine information of the kind that commissioners and deci-sion-makers need for orientation and initial planning is easily access-ible. The days when only specialist analysts had access to information and summary statistical products about local health care and other population outcomes is no longer the case. The sources below can be used to complement any other local knowledge- and literature-based evidence sources. The commissioner and decision-maker adds value by applying the relevant health information in context and through re-sulting actions.

Examples of general sources:

- *PHE Statistics*[2] Contain information across many themes, in-cluding summary profiles for local areas in England, premature mortality, and a range of condition-specific topics (e.g. stroke, diabetes, heart disease, kidney disease, cancers, liver disease)
- *NHS Digital*[1] Contains a range of health-service outcomes.
- *Prescribing data*[4] Contains general practice prescribing data at local level and national level.
- *Mortality statistics*[5]
- *Birth statistics*[6]
- *Local products*. For example Joint Strategic Needs Assessment (JSNA) resource in England.[7,8] This can provide a more in-depth lens on local priorities.

Some sources are accessible on an organizational need-to-use basis only rather than via general access. For these you will need guidance from your information analysts to advise what is feasible and available for your organization. Examples of these sources are:

- *Local hospital activity* ('Hospital Episode Statistics' or 'Secondary Uses Service'). Contains accident and emergency, inpatients and outpatient data.[9,10]
- *Contracting or commissioning datasets* (nationally or locally defined).

c. *Local context and pathways knowledge.* This is knowledge of the local care pathways and their interdependencies. It helps you to gauge the feasibility and degree of support from local networks. This is the real-life backdrop for your decision-making.

You could think of it as a *'Trio of commissioning knowledge'* for the commissioner to try and gather. Anyone who has practised in this arena can tell you that ignoring any one of these areas makes for less informed and less confident decision-making; or that just using one of these perspectives whilst ignoring the other two can make leadership efforts for health much more difficult to achieve.

Health information themes

As with evidence-based sources from research studies, there is no single repository of all the health information sources you might need to inform your decision-making, and even if there were, it would be out-of-date quite soon. However, the general themes that the data collections fall into are quite consistent, which are:

- *Demographics* (e.g. population size, age and sex structure, deprivation indices);
- *Service usage and access to services* (e.g. GP practices, hospital and mental health services);
- *Outcomes* (mortality, morbidity and patient experience);
- *Wider contextual information about the population* (e.g. risk-factor prevalence, environment, crime, education, etc);
- *Specific conditions* (routine or ad hoc collections about cancers, strokes, and liver disease data, etc).

Again, the question you pose is pertinent as it helps you to seek the information you need rather than that which is presented to you, or if something is presented to you, you will know whether it is relevant to what you need.

Making sense of economic evaluations

You will now have a feel for the key areas of use of information for health services commissioning and decision-making, and the general themes of the data available. The focus of this chapter has been about the application of information rather than on specific information sources, however there follows a specific mention of the information from economic evaluations at this point because although the concepts are not difficult once grasped, they may initially take a little more orientation to appreciate than some of the other perhaps more easy to digest statistics in health intelligence (such as incidence, activity data, or deaths).

Information from economic evaluations is another type of information that commissioners will come across. For example, it is included as part of the reviewed information in national guidance documents in England from the National Institute of Health and Care Excellence (NICE).[11] When available, such information is most directly relevant to the planning and prioritization aspects of the commissioning cycle. As with other types of health information, that from economic evaluations should be used to inform decision-making, rather than dictating a decision.

Economic evaluation can be defined as the 'comparative analysis of alternative courses of action in terms of both their costs and consequences.'[12] They are structured attempts to determine whether an intervention is an efficient use of societal resources. This line of enquiry is clearly relevant for healthcare commissioning, where the consequences (health outcomes) and costs (from a finite resource) matter a lot.

The conduct of economic evaluations and health economics as a whole is a disciplinary field in its own right, and for more in-depth exploration of the development of economic evaluation measures, assumptions, uses, and limitations there are dedicated texts.[12,13] The following is an orientation to terminology as it is an aspect of health intelligence awareness needed by the commissioner.

In essence, economic evaluations look at what you get for a particular cost. Decision-makers could just compare outcomes (e.g. which alternative works better?) but that would not take into account costs. And if they compared only the costs (e.g. which one is cheaper?), that would not take account of whether health outcomes were achieved, which is the point of healthcare commissioning. So health economic evaluation techniques are of interest to decision-makers because they aim to take account of both costs and outcomes and compare alternative strategies. Information from economic evaluations may originate from studies in their own right or may be part of an intervention study.

It is helpful at this point to also note two useful terms that you may hear being used in relation to the distribution and use of resources. These are allocative efficiency and technical efficiency. In the healthcare context allocative efficiency refers to achieving the best value for money or optimal distribution of resources across all the many possible programmes of care. Technical efficiency is concerned with achieving the best value for money out of a specific programme of care, or other agreed objective, when the programme budget or objective has already been accepted.

For orientation, three main types of economic evaluation information will be described. These are cost-effectiveness analysis, cost-utility analysis, and cost-benefit analysis. Note that sometimes in conversation the term cost-effectiveness is used generally to mean information from cost-effectiveness analysis or from cost-utility analysis and you will have to work out from the context whether both are meant or not.

Cost-effectiveness analysis

Cost-effectiveness analysis (CEA) aims to address the question, 'what is the best way of achieving outcome X?'. It is useful in scenarios where the objective has already been agreed (for example to reduce hypertension in the population or to reduce pain in chronic arthritis), and information is needed about the most efficient means of achieving the result. CEA therefore addresses technical efficiency questions.

The measures are described in terms of cost per unit of effect, where the effect is measured in natural units such as reduction in blood pressure as measured in millimetres of mercury, or the number of pain-free days. So if for example a drug to modify the course of rheumatoid arthritis costs £55 per pain-free day and another therapy costs £300 per pain-free day, then the first option has a lower cost–effectiveness ratio and is deemed more cost-effective on that measure.

Clearly, such statistics are dependent on the quality of the data on effectiveness of interventions and services, and most studies would therefore have sensitivity analyses (to test the extent that any changes in assumptions affect the results).

Cost-utility analysis

Cost-utility analysis (CUA) aims to address the question: 'What effective things should healthcare provide overall?' With CEA, different areas of healthcare cannot be compared directly because the outcomes may be measured in different units. For example, it is difficult to compare the value of a reduction in blood pressure with a week's worth of pain-free days from rheumatoid arthritis. CUA attempts to overcome this difficulty by measuring outcomes using a common unit, called a 'utility'.

The utility outcome measure takes into account both the quality and duration of life, resulting in a measure known as a quality-adjusted life year (QALY). This estimates the years of life remaining for a person following a particular intervention, and applies a weighting based on quality of life (on a 0 to 1 scale). The quality of life component of the QALY is assessed using standardized methods (commonly the EQ-5D for adults is used which covers a range of themes including mobility, pain, mental distress, and ability to carry out activities of daily life).[11] With the QALY statistic, a year of life in perfect health is represented by a QALY of 1. A year of less than perfect health has a QALY between zero and 1, and death has a QALY of zero. Combined with information on cost, the resulting CUA measure is given as a cost per QALY.

The cost per QALY is thus another type of cost-effectiveness ratio, albeit using a utility (the QALY) as the outcome measure instead of a natural unit as with the CEA technique. Usually the cost per QALY statistic is used to describe the extra cost per extra unit of health effect compared to a current alternative, and so is referred to as an 'incremental cost-effectiveness ratio'. For example, the cost per QALY for total hip replacement has been estimated at £7,182 per QALY compared with no surgery[14] and the cost per QALY for angioplasty has been estimated at £9,241 per QALY compared with medical management.[15]

So the main advantages of CUA over CEA are that different courses of action can be compared using a common currency, and quality of life can be taken into account. CUA can therefore help explore allocative efficiency (how best to apportion our resources across the many different competing options to maximize overall benefit), and can make the opportunity costs more apparent. Within a programme of care, CUA measures can also be used to address technical efficiency.

A big practical limitation is that CUAs are time consuming to produce, so the information might not be available for all the topics you might need to compare. Clearly also, issues of valuing health and life with a single summary measure necessarily includes a variety of subjective assessments, so the transparency of methods used for assessing utility is important for interpretation and use.

Another practical point to note before we leave CUA is the idea of a cost-effectiveness threshold. Although in theory it is possible to compile a league table of cost per QALYs to compare alternatives for value for money, in practice the comparative information might not be available so a 'threshold' approach is often used to guide whether a cost per QALY indicates value for money or not.[16] For example, if a notional threshold of £30,000 per QALY is used, then interventions with a cost per QALY below the threshold would be considered cost-effective and suitable for further consideration for funding, whereas interventions with a cost per QALY above the threshold would not be deemed cost-effective and so are less suitable for funding, other things being equal. (Sometimes the guiding threshold is described as a range, for example £20,000 to £30,000 per QALY). That is not to say that higher cost per QALY items are not funded, as there may be other factors that are taken into account in the decision-making, but the cost-effectiveness component is clearer. This of course leads to debates about what is an appropriate threshold for cost-effectiveness in health and healthcare, and there is unlikely to be a black and white answer to that quest that will be universally acceptable.[17] If a guide is needed, commissioners might refer to a range described by an existing authority e.g. NICE.[11] In practice, a commissioner would also have a range of other factors to consider in addition to cost-effectiveness in their deliberations about whether to fund something or not (see Chapter 10). The main thing is that any thresholds are pragmatic and if used as part of making recommendations for funding something, or not, they should be explicit.

With these practical caveats in mind, CUAs continue to be produced in practice in the health service arena. Where they are available, they are another type of comparative health information for the decision-maker, particularly for the planning and prioritization phases of commissioning. As with all other health information, it is a source of decision support rather than a deterministic tool.

Cost–benefit analysis

The concept of cost–benefit analysis (CBA) was mooted before the development of CUA, but you may still come across it in healthcare situations. The concept aims to address allocative efficiency questions ('what should healthcare provide?') and so can inform scenarios where there is an overall budget that can be allocated across different competing options but it is still unclear which objectives to pursue.

Costs and benefits are both measured using the same monetary units (for example pounds sterling). The analysis gives a net economic difference when the costs of the proposed scheme are subtracted from the benefits to assess whether the benefits exceed the costs.[11] The principle is to only do things where the benefits exceed costs and not do things where costs exceed benefits. If there are several things where benefit exceeds cost they can be compared to help inform decision-making.

With CBA, a wide range of societal costs can be included, not just health-care costs (e.g. days of work lost, cost of travel). The outcomes or 'benefits' are conventionally given a monetary value using recognized methods to es-timate this.[18]

Clearly there can be difficulties with a concept that values health using monetary terms only, so the transparency of methods of attributing such benefits used in CBA is important for interpretation of the findings. Because of the difficulties with valuing life and health in monetary terms only, healthcare cost–benefit analysis tends only to be used in economic evaluation of capital projects and other structural items (e.g. buildings and equipment) rather than on direct patient care.[18]

Other summary statistics with a bigger picture spirit

You might also come across other statistics or analyses which aim to give a bigger picture awareness of the impact of an intervention. Examples are the 'number needed to treat',[19] population impact number,[20] and return on in-vestment estimates.[21] When available, these also add to the information for decision-making, and the general tack of making sense of the information they contribute and using that to inform the planning and assessment of services remains relevant.

Round-up

No matter how good our information systems and their data analysing infrastructures are, it will always be important to frame a question be-fore interrogating or requesting data. Good questions help to build our knowledge of the issues in order to find solutions so that the information gained can contribute to improving the way we understand, plan, prioritize, and evaluate care. With the 'three uses' model in mind, whatever the range of information, technology solutions, and datasets available, they are potential tools and ingredients to help answer relevant questions for decision-making.

Do not be put off by its apparent simplicity. Next time it is not clear why an exercise to produce information has been requested, why not use this model to challenge each other. Try it!

Reflection

Think about an occasion in the last two months when you requested some health information. Was it clear to you from the outset what question(s) the health information would be helping you to answer?

If yes, was it to understand the nature and extent of the problem, plan a way of addressing the problem, or to find out if things were moving in the right direction?

If you did it again now, what would you do differently, if anything?

References

1. NHS Digital. Data and information. Available at: https://digital.nhs.uk/data-and-information
2. Public Health England. Statistics at PHE. Available at: https://www.gov.uk/government/organisations/public-health-england/about/statistics
3. Oxford English Dictionary. Oxford University Press. Available at: https://en.oxforddictionaries.com/english
4. NHS Digital. Practice level prescribing data. Available at: https://digital.nhs.uk/data-and-information/publications/statistical/practice-level-prescribing-data
5. Office for National Statistics. Death registrations summary tables – England and Wales. July 2018 release. Available at: https://www.ons.gov.uk/peoplepopulationandcommunity/birthsdeathsandmarriages/deaths/datasets/deathregistrationssummarytablesenglandandwalesreferencetables
6. Office for National Statistics. Births in England and Wales summary tables. July 2018 release. Available at: https://www.ons.gov.uk/peoplepopulationandcommunity/birthsdeathsandmarriages/livebirths/datasets/birthsummarytables
7. Department of Health. Joint strategic needs assessment and joint health and wellbeing strategies explained. Gateway reference 16731. December 2011.

Available at: https://assets.publishing.service.gov.uk/government/uploads/system/uploads/attachment_data/file/215261/dh_131733.pdf

8. Department of Health. Statutory guidance on joint strategic needs assessments and joint health and wellbeing strategies. Gateway reference 18840. March 2013. Available at: https://assets.publishing.service.gov.uk/government/uploads/system/uploads/attachment_data/file/277012/Statutory-Guidance-on-Joint-Strategic-Needs-Assessments-and-Joint-Health-and-Wellbeing-Strategies-March-20131.pdf

9. NHS Digital. Hospital episode statistics (HES). Available at: https://digital.nhs.uk/data-and-information/data-tools-and-services/data-services/hospital-episode-statistics

10. NHS Digital. Secondary Uses Service (SUS). Available at: https://digital.nhs.uk/services/secondary-uses-service-sus

11. NICE. Developing NICE guidelines: the manual. Process and methods [PMG20]. Updated October 2018. Available at: https://www.nice.org.uk/process/pmg20/chapter/incorporating-economic-evaluation#the-role-of-economics-in-guideline-development

12. Drummond M, Sculpher M, Caxton K, Stoddart GL, Torrance GW. *Methods for the Economic Evaluation of Health Care Programmes.* Fourth edition). Oxford Medical Publications, 2015.

13. Mooney G. *Economics, Medicine and Health Care.* Third edition. Financial Times Management, 2003.

14. Fordham R, Skinner J, Wang X, Nolan J. The economic benefit of hip replacement: a 5-year follow-up of costs and outcomes in the Exeter Primary Outcomes Study. *BMJ Open* 2012;2:e000752. doi: 10.1136/bmjopen-2011-000752

15. Bravo Vergel Y, Palmer S, Asseburg C, Fenwick E, de Belder M, Abrams K et al. Is primary angioplasty cost effective in the UK? Results of a comprehensive decision analysis. *Heart* 2007;93(10):1238–1243.

16. NICE. Guide to the methods of technology appraisal 2013. PMG9. April 2013. Available at: https://www.nice.org.uk/process/pmg9/chapter/the-reference-case#framework-for-estimating-clinical-and-cost-effectiveness

17. Appleby J. Crossing the line: NICE's value for money threshold. *BMJ* 2016;352:i1336.

18. York Health Economics Consortium. Cost-Benefit Analysis [online]. 2016. Available at: https://www.yhec.co.uk/glossary/cost-benefit-analysis/

19. York Health Economics Consortium. Number Needed to Treat. 2016. Available at: https://www.yhec.co.uk/glossary/number-needed-to-treat/

20. Heller RF, Dobson AJ. Disease impact number and population impact number: population perspectives to measures of risk and benefit. *BMJ* 2000;2014;321(7266): 950–953.

21. York Health Economics Consortium. Return on Investment [online]. 2016. Available at: https://www.yhec.co.uk/glossary/return-on-investment

PART II

ENABLING LEADERSHIP FOR A POPULATION APPROACH TO HEALTH SERVICES DECISION-MAKING

9
Population Approach to All Levels of Commissioning and Health Service Decision-Making

This chapter is a bird's eye view of the further synergistic links between a population approach and different levels of health service planning and decision-making.

Chapter 3 has already described key vantage points and the importance of taking a population approach to commissioning. To recap, this includes a needs-led and evidence-seeking approach to understanding the bigger picture of health, effective preventive opportunities, inequalities in access and outcomes, and a consideration of the whole care pathway. It also described how the relationship between commissioning processes and striving for population health gain is an overlapping endeavour. This interconnecting relationship remains relevant whatever the policies and structural arrangements of the day with respect to where health-service decisions are made, and where the population health skills for commissioning reside in the health system. This functional relationship is not only relevant at the day-to-day level but also at the system level. The close working of commissioning skills and healthcare public health functions (HCPH) has been recognized earlier (Chapters 3 and 5). They are co-dependent and synergistic because commissioning is concerned with securing effective services for the population, and HCPH practice (sometimes called health services improvement) is concerned with improving health outcomes through the effectiveness of health services.[1,2,3] From a commissioning perspective, work in this area can also be seen as commissioning for health gain.

The health gain focus therefore complements some of the more transactional aspects of commissioning and potentiates the value of commissioning in general. The value of such inputs at the practical day-to-day level of service commissioning work in the English system has been recognized.[4,5] What has been less well articulated in the practical literature perhaps is that this synergy is not only relevant for commissioning related

Commissioning and a Population Approach to Health Services Decision-Making. Julie Sin, Oxford University Press (2020). © Oxford University Press. DOI: 10.1093/oso/9780198840732.001.0001

activities at the day-to-day level but it is also relevant for health services decision-making in general. In essence, one cannot commission properly without taking a population approach.

Main points to be familiar with ...

- Pragmatically, healthcare commissioning activities can be described at different levels; these can be considered as strategic, tactical, and operational levels.
- A population approach to decision-making is *integral* to all these levels of commissioning decisions.

Population approach and health services commissioning in unison at all levels of commissioning activity

From a bird's-eye view, the activities and decision-making points in commissioning can pragmatically be considered as strategic, tactical, and operational level activities (see Figure 9.1). Strategic-level considerations relate to governance and direction-setting activities. These responsibilities tend to be continuous in nature. Tactical-level considerations relate to activities that directly enable strategic objectives e.g. activities to prioritize resources, or a major service review across the population. These responsibilities and projects may be time limited but their alignment to strategic purpose is clear. Operational activities in this context refer to day-to-day 'business as usual' aspects of the commissioning cycle. These responsibilities tend to be more transactional, though they should also directly or indirectly contribute to achieving the overall strategic objectives.

Figure 9.1 also offers examples of matters and decisions requiring a population perspective across the range of strategic, tactical, and operational commissioning levels. The population approach, represented here by HCPH (though it is recognized that these skills can be distributed widely across a health system) is clearly integral to all levels of commissioning activity.

Although HCPH practice can help to steer this input, for a truly disseminated population approach to health service decision-making, a wide and

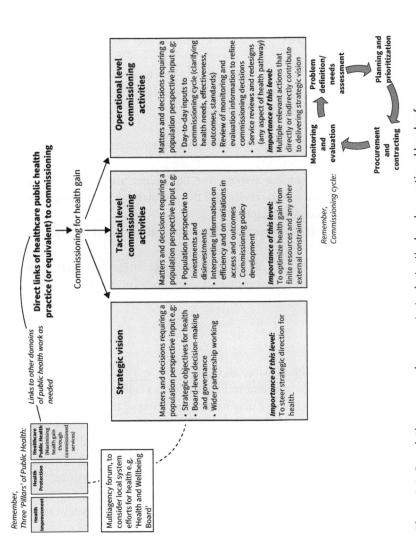

Figure 9.1 Population approach across strategic, tactical and operational levels of commissioning activities

multidisciplinary range of colleagues working in the commissioning arena need to have awareness of population perspectives to decision-making and the different levels of activity that it is part of.

Uses of the model

The model in Figure 9.1 can be used to provide practical orientation and enable thinking about the population perspective to health services decision-making at a system level. It can be used to:

- show that a population approach has an underpinning role at all levels of commissioning activity;
- develop commissioning systems (or equivalent strategic planning process to secure health services for the population) with population health gain as a core principle;
- support leadership in commissioning for health gain across the system.

For further interest, Box 9.1 illustrates how a population approach feeds into many levels of health services planning and decision-making.

Practicalities

Healthcare public health activity and health services commissioning have been shown as separate functions in Figure 9.1; this is illustrative. In some integrated arrangements, there may be no separation of the two functions as they operate as a general commissioning function within a common organization (for example as may be the case with some specialized services and screening programmes, and as was the general case with commissioning arrangements before 2013 and in some evolving systems since).

Given the breadth of the commissioning arena, a wide range of participants are likely to need to be familiar with a population approach in their commissioning contributions. HCPH skills and experience can be a key enabler of the approach because of its existing practice in this area. As a health service commissioner, after gaining a working orientation of the scope of services that your organization commissions, it will be useful to find out whether HCPH support is already part of your organization or whether you need to establish these links. It would be a useful starting point for enabling

Box 9.1 How the population health gain approach is incorporated as part of health services decision-making at many levels

Consider the following scenarios to illustrate:

Commissioning organization X wants to commission an acute stroke service for its residents. A multidisciplinary team works on this. To understand and build the practical case for this they actively seek input about the size of the problem; the estimated health need (problems which have an effective solution); what the current evidence says about effective opportunities to reduce the impact of the condition; any cost-effectiveness information; outcomes such a service should monitor; and any available information on inequities of access and outcomes of services. As part of this basic case building they also consider wider service interdependencies (with rehabilitation, primary care, and links to general care), and any particular features of their local patient flows (for example if a motorway or natural feature such as a river means the population tends to travel in particular directions more than others).

This takes a bit of effort but it makes it easier for them to consider the merits of the stroke service proposal when it comes to deciding which investments can be supported in the coming year. Their process for assessing proposals for investments already explicitly includes health gain as a key factor to be considered. Decision-taking at the board level, if needed, is also easier because the proposal is in keeping with the organization's strategic priorities. In addition, the board configuration already includes a member with a lead role for ensuring that population effectiveness and reducing health inequalities is taken into account. There are further practical steps involving contracting, but the service is successfully commissioned for the population. 'Strategic, tactical, and operational' commissioning activities were brought into play and all encompassed a population health gain perspective.

Commissioning organization Y wants to review its commissioning of local mental health services because of local service sustainability issues. Work begins to assess the practical case and they actively seek input about the many operational-level commissioning details needed (just as commissioner X did in the previous example). They soon realize that the topic content is more complex and the group of health conditions involved is more heterogeneous than a simple service location for a single condition. They reflect that the whole local system perspective will be pertinent and that maintaining a population health gain focus is a crucial part of this. Not only would the latter help to secure potentially better health outcomes from these services, but it would also help as a means of engaging support from clinicians, patients and carers, and other stakeholders.

They reflected that their board structure already included responsibility for considering effectiveness and inequalities, and that their prioritization processes took health gain into account. They had also previously contributed to compiling the local joint strategic needs assessment on mental health needs in the area and had learned from that experience. With their background work they were better prepared for local stakeholder scrutiny on the options. Through further understanding of local context and engagement of stakeholders they also understood more about interdependent services (e.g. services for people with other overlapping health and care needs). Though these enabling steps took many months, a new service was commissioned for the population with monitoring for ongoing effectiveness in place. 'Strategic, tactical, and operational' commissioning activities had been brought into play and all had encompassed a population health gain perspective.

and building up your local resources for a population approach to health service decision-making.

Summary

The policy contexts of population health and health services commissioning must be coherent with each other in order to secure health gain through commissioned services. They may or may not easily dovetail with each other as national and local arrangements evolve, but it is one of the challenges for healthcare leaders to navigate in the system they find themselves in.

> **Reflection**
>
> Where is the local HCPH support to local health services commissioning?
> What are the strengths and weaknesses of the arrangement? What needs
> to change to strengthen this relationship?

References

1. NHS. Health Education England. What is public health? Available at: https://www.healthcareers.nhs.uk/working-health/working-public-health/what-public-health
2. House of Commons. House of Commons Health Committee. Public Health Post-2013. HC 140. 2016.
3. Faculty of Public Health. Good Public Health Practice Framework 2016. Available at: https://www.fph.org.uk/media/1304/good-public-health-practice-framework_-2016_final.pdf
4. Department of Health. Healthcare Public Health Advice to Clinical Commissioning Groups: Guidance to support the provision of healthcare public health advice to CCG. Gateway number 17804. June 2012.
5. Public Health England. Core offer: The Healthcare Public Health Advice Service to Clinical Commissioning Groups. Gateway number 2017228. August 2017.

10

Prioritization of Investments and Disinvestments in Healthcare

A Conceptual Toolkit

This chapter looks at the key elements to have in place to enable coherent decision-making about prioritization of investments and disinvestments of finite resources in healthcare.

> ### Main points to be familiar with ...
>
> - Core elements of a coherent decision-making process.
> - A 'prioritization tool' you can adapt, to gather and sift information.
> - Types of prioritization scenarios to recognize.

This is a big topic, as anyone who has ever been involved in prioritization knows, and there will be many particular facets that you will need to think about the handling of as you venture down this process in practice. That said, once thought through, there are few if any of these issues that cannot be considered within a well-constructed overarching ethical commissioning framework. This chapter gives the crucial bearings you will need to construct a prioritization approach and get you started. Beyond that you will need to practise your own 'good enough' approach, learn and refine over time to perfect a process that works to help you to do the job effectively. Ideally, each organization should have a version of this overall process. Ask about it at your organization. If you cannot uncover a coherent process, ask questions or ask if you can help to develop one.

At its best a prioritization process is a transparent, consistent, and pragmatic attempt to make reasonable decisions with the information available. From experience, once a good enough process has been put together, it is best approached as a perennial 'do and refine' process that is owned by the organization, and each year's learning continues to enhance the process.

Commissioning and a Population Approach to Health Services Decision-Making. Julie Sin, Oxford University Press (2020). © Oxford University Press. DOI: 10.1093/oso/9780198840732.001.0001

The synopsis in this chapter is an all-in-one-place guide about three key components that are needed to enable an effective priority setting and decision-making system. It is based on over fifteen years' experience of developing and seeing this in action within local and sub-regional levels of health services commissioning, using 'do and refine' processes to improve with new learning.

Within the chapter there is a description about a prioritization tool (sometimes called a prioritization matrix) to assist the information gathering and information sifting part of the process. This is followed by further orientation to the practical processes of such prioritization and decision-making. The chapter then completes by acknowledging the importance of having an ethical framework and recognizing the challenges that decision-making for populations sometimes presents.

A process for understanding choices and risks

Not everything that is effective is cost-effective, and not everything that is cost-effective is affordable. Furthermore, using resources for one choice means those resources are not available for something else ('opportunity costs'). An organization that is securing or 'buying' services for its population will need to make decisions about how to make best use of finite resources, in meeting the needs of its population.

To support this effort, organizations will need to develop a workable prioritization process for making investment and disinvestment decisions. In reality, this process will involve a combination of evidence and judgements and there needs to be explicit opportunity to take account of both. A 'good enough' process will help to:

- understand the balance of benefits and risks of different choices, including opportunity costs;
- promote consistency and transparency of the principles and processes used;
- communicate about the decisions made;
- be a continuous learning process for future iterations.

The approach can be used to prioritize the proposals for investments, potential disinvestments, existing resources, or a mixture of these, depending on the scenario. When set up, the principles, processes, and any facilitative tool used will help with the annual commissioning round for investment and disinvestment decisions.

Core elements of a coherent prioritization process

Good decisions depend on having a relevant frame of reference, being able to gather relevant information, and having a system to review it and take responsibility for the decisions. In practice, a coherent prioritization process is enabled by the following three core elements:

Guiding principles for priority setting

This is sometimes called an 'Ethical Framework for Priority Setting'. This sets out overarching principles for commissioning decisions. They apply to all types of commissioning decisions, whether they are proposals for service developments or individual funding requests. The principles are remarkably consistent across health commissioners e.g. clinical and cost-effectiveness, opportunity cost, balancing needs of populations with needs of individuals. This is covered in more detail later in the chapter.

Use of a prioritization tool or format

This is about gathering relevant information in a consistent format and assessing the information. Such a tool usually provides two purposes:

(i) a *common format* to gather relevant information about each proposal and,

(ii) *common criteria* that each proposal will be assessed against.

The criteria used reflect the organization's guiding principles for priority setting and typically include practical criteria about health gain, cost, and risk. Often a pragmatic and peer agreed 'scoring and weighting' system is used to help rank the various proposals in an initial order for discussion.

The tool facilitates decision-making but does not replace the corporate responsibility to sense check and formally make decisions about competing needs for resources.

Coherent decision-making process

The process for decision-making needs to be clear from the outset. In its simplest form there will need to be a decision-making body to ratify and take responsibility for the decisions (e.g. a governing body or a board-level structure). For smooth running, organizations may have in place some kind of priority setting group to review the information, propose an order of priority, and make considered recommendations to the decision-making group. This overall process therefore allows opportunities for sense-checking stages to be built in.

To look at these concepts further, the most tangible place to start is to look at the prioritization tool element. The following section describes how a prioritization tool can contribute to the process. The basic principles can be adapted for your own use.

A prioritization tool

One of the main advantages of using a prioritization tool is that it helps to make the assessment of risks and benefits of a proposal explicit. It helps to compare the relative merits of different proposals more consistently, and facilitates some initial ranking across proposals for further discussion. It is an *aid* to prioritization, rather than a deterministic tool, and it does not replace the need for decision-making processes. The responsibility to make ethical judgements taking into account health gain, risks, and contextual considerations remains with the accountable body such as the board, unless explicitly delegated to another body.

The common criteria that will be used to assess each proposal are agreed at the start of the process. Typically these aim to identify the main risks and benefits of each proposal. Each proposal for investment (or disinvestment if the process is being run that way around) is thus assessed against a consistent list of criteria. To assist the process, the criteria per se could also be the basis of constructing a common format for submitting information about proposals.

To illustrate, Table 10.1 is an example of criteria used to assess proposals for funding. It is based on a real-life tool that has been used by a health services commissioning organization in England.[1] (You may have your own local tool for such purposes or may choose to develop one suitable for your local needs. In this example, its development had been informed by local and national practice,[2,3] then further tailored for local use via a multidisciplinary workshop to gain consensus for the approach.)

In the example, criteria are across five categories, namely strategic fit, health gain, risks, financial information, and deliverability. Each proposal is considered in turn. A score is given for each of the criteria and a total score is derived for each proposal. Prompts and guidance can be used to help allocate scores against each of the criteria (see Table 10.2 later in the chapter from which the criteria in Table 10.1 are drawn). The exercise results in a range of scores for the competing proposals to inform the decision-making discussions.

The weighting across the categories is pragmatic and peer agreed. You will see that in Table 10.1 the relative weightings out of a hundred across the categories are distributed in the ratio of 10:40:25:15:10. These may be balanced differently in different organizations and may be amended over time even within an organization. The importance is that there is some deliberation and overall consensus on the weightings to be used as part of the tool for that cycle.

You can develop your own local format and weightings suitable for local use. For example, you might choose to focus on health gain aspects only, as that may be sufficient for your situation. In the example given, the commissioning organization has also chosen to make explicit some of the risks and practicalities of each proposal within the tool. From experience, this is a reasonable idea as decision-makers spend much time in reality considering the risks as well as the health gain in their deliberations. This type of format explicitly looks at the effects on health gain and at risks of inaction, and is an attempt to prevent inadvertently not considering one or the other in the heat of the moment. The main thing is for the organization and local stakeholders to feel it is helpful and workable for them.

As there might be many proposals to work though as part of the process, keeping track of the deliberations is important. Box 10.1 is a sample format that can be used to summarize findings from each proposal. As well as the total score for each proposal, the values for each component category (e.g. health gain, risk, etc.) are clear as well. Such a format thus allows flexibility

Table 10.1 Example of criteria in a prioritization tool and weightings

Criteria to consider for each proposal	Score range for criterion (x scaling factor)	Scores (weighting of category out of 100)
Strategic fit		
Proposal contributes to a strategic goal (or another goal which the organization has committed to).	1 to 5 (x2)	
		Subtotal (__/10)
Health Gain		
Strength of the evidence that proposed intervention/service has a positive effect*	1 to 5 (x2)	
Size of the clinical benefit	1 to 5 (x1)	
Number of people to benefit	1 to 5 (x1)	
Patient acceptability	1 to 5 (x1)	
Quality of life	1 to 5 (x1)	
Impact on access and equity	1 to 5 (x1)	
Contribution to preventing ill health and/or further need for health or care services	1 to 5 (x1)	
		Subtotal (__/40)
Risks (if activity does not go ahead)		
Risk of not reaching national/local targets	1 to 5 (x1)	
Clinical risk	1 to 5 (x1)	
Financial risk	1 to 5 (x1)	
Political/reputational risk	1 to 5 (x1)	
Impact on other services	1 to 5 (x1)	
		Subtotal (__/25)
Financial costs and savings		
Cost of service (per annum)	1 to 5 (x2)	
Return on investment (evidence of)	1 to 5 (x1)	
		Subtotal (__/15)
Deliverability		
Speed of delivering the project	1 to 5 (x0.5)	
Ease of delivering	1 to 5 (x0.5)	
Initiation costs (£)	1 to 5 (x0.5)	
Number of people to set up service.	1 to 5 (x0.5)	
		Subtotal (__/10)
TOTAL score for each proposal		__/100

(*Source: Data from Prioritisation tool, NHS Eastern Cheshire CCG[1]*)
* Anything shown to be unsafe or with no positive effect through these criteria should not be assessed any further as part of the commissioning round. For prompts and guidance to help allocate scores for each criteria, see Table 10.2 which shows the full matrix that Table 10.1 is derived from.

Table 10.2 Example prioritization tool ('matrix')

		Score 1	Score 2	Score 3	Score 4	Score 5	Weighting	Proposal A	Proposal B	etc....
Strategic fit	**Strategic fit.** Extent that proposals contribute to strategic goals	Unknown or no contribution	Some contribution	Moderate contribution	Significant contribution	Major contribution	x 2			
							Subtotal	/10	/10	
Health gain	**Strength of evidence.** The highest level of evidence that the proposed intervention/service has a positive effect?	Lower level e.g. case-studies, anecdotal	Low to modest evidence e.g. descriptive study with no comparison group	Moderate evidence e.g. descriptive study with a comparison group	At least one well conducted randomized trial	Meta-analysis/ systematic review	x 2			
	Magnitude of the clinical benefit to the individual if it works	Negligible (e.g. <10% cf. cure)	Some improvement	Moderate improvement (e.g. 50% cf cure)	Significant improvement	Very significant gain in health (e.g. near cure)	x1			
	Number of people that would benefit*	<20 (less than 1 in 10,000)	20 to 100 (1 to 5 in 10,000)	101 to 1,000 (0.51 to 5 in 1,000)	1,001 to 5,000 (5 to 25 in 1,000)	Over 5,000 (>25 in 1,000)	x1			
	Patient acceptability e.g. of service location or method of treatment	Patients consider it unacceptable	Patients consider it somewhat unacceptable	Patients have a neutral opinion on the whole	Patients consider it somewhat positively	Patients consider it very positively	x1			
	Quality of life e.g. disability reduction, independence, pain reduction, social relationships	No improvement	Some improvement	Moderate improvement	Significant improvement	Compelling life changing improvement	x1			

	No effect or not applicable	Some effect	Moderate effect	Significant effect	Major effect	x1
Access and equity. Proposal enables equitable access to healthcare or reduces inequities in outcomes	No effect or not applicable	Some effect	Moderate effect	Significant effect	Major effect	x1
Prevention. Proposal reduces ill health and/ or need for further health and care services	No contribution or not applicable	Some contribution	Moderate contribution	Significant contribution	Major contribution	x1
				Subtotal /40	/40	
Risks						
Risk of not achieving targets. What is the impact on national or local targets if proposal does not go ahead	Minimum impact	Some risk and impact on ability to achieve targets	Moderate risk and impact on ability to achieve targets	Significant risk and impact on ability to achieve targets	Major risk and impact on ability to achieve targets	x1
Clinical risk. What is the risk if this service is not implemented?	Minimum impact	Some risk and impact if project does not go ahead	Moderate risk and impact if project does not go ahead	Significant risk and impact if project does not go ahead	Major risk and impact if project does not go ahead	x1
Financial risk. What is the risk if the project does not go ahead?	Minimum impact	Some risk and impact if project does not go ahead	Moderate risk and impact if project does not go ahead	Significant risk and impact if project does not go ahead	Major risk and impact if project does not go ahead	x1
Reputational risk. What is the risk if the project does not go ahead?	Minimum impact	Some risk and impact if project does not go ahead	Moderate risk and impact if project does not go ahead	Significant risk and impact if project does not go ahead	Major risk and impact if project does not go ahead	x1

(Continued)

Table 10.2 (Continued)

		Score 1	Score 2	Score 3	Score 4	Score 5	Weighting	Proposal A	Proposal B	etc....
	Impact of proposal on other services or other provider(s) if it goes ahead	Clear negative impact on provider(s)	Some negative impact on other providers	No impact on other service providers	Some positive impact on other providers	Service gap identified, will assist other service providers	x1			
							Subtotal	/25	/25	
Financial costs and savings	Cost of service per annum	> £500,000	£250,000 to £500,000	£100,000 to £250,000	£30,000 to £100000	< £30,000	x 2			
	Return on investment. Evidence base for a positive return on investment	No financial return on investment, or lower level evidence e.g. opinion only	Minimal evidence e.g. descriptive study	Modest evidence e.g. descriptive study with plausible likelihood	Good evidence e.g. descriptive study with comparison group	Significant evidence e.g. intervention study with validated methods	x 1			
							Subtotal	/15	/15	
Delivery	Speed of delivery. How quickly can the project be delivered?	> 1 year or unknown	6 months to 1 year	3 to 6 months	1 to 3 months	Within 1 month	x 0.5			
	Ease of delivery of this type of project	Highly complex project with little experience of delivery	Some complexity and experience of delivery	Moderate experience of delivery	Significant experience of completing this type of project before	This type of project can be undertaken as part of business as usual	x 0.5			

Initiation costs (£) e.g. pump priming and project costs	> £500,000	> £250,000 to £500,000	> £100,000 to £250,000	£30,000 to £100,000	< £30,000	x 0.5
People resources. How many people will be engaged in setting up the project?	More than 5 full time staff for duration of project, or unknown	2 to 4 staff full time	1 member of staff full time	1 member of staff working 2 to 4 days per week	1 member of staff working < 1 day per week	x 0.5

Subtotal /10   /10

TOTAL __/100

(*Source: Data from 'Prioritisation tool', NHS Eastern Cheshire CCG*[1])
*Based on population circa 200,000.

Box 10.1 **Example summary sheet for each proposal**

For use by the prioritization panel. Use a separate sheet for each proposal. Guidance for scoring is in the prioritization matrix tool agreed for this round.

Title of proposal:

Date:

Reference number:

A. Categories and Scores

Strategic fit	(Max.10)
Health gain (Quality and Effectiveness)	(Max.40)
Risks	(Max.25)
Financial costs and savings	(Max.15)
'Deliverability'	(Max.10)
TOTAL	(Max. 100)

B. Summary of Benefits and Risks
These can be compared with existing arrangements if relevant.

Main Benefit(s) of the proposal

Main Risk(s) if proposal does not go ahead

Any other comments

(Source: Data from NHS Eastern Cheshire CCG[1])

for the health gain component or the risks to be understood separately if needed.

To a pure mathematician it may seem a little unsatisfactory to use numbers in this way, as the numbers being aggregated come from an ordinal or 'ranking' scale (a scale of measurement in which the higher the number the greater the value but the size of distance between consecutive units is not necessarily the same), rather than from an 'interval scale' of measurement (in which the higher the number the greater the value, *and* the difference between two consecutive numbers is the same size).[4] The context here is important though, as decision-making is a multidimensional set of considerations and the tool is trying to help make this explicit. Any such tool is a pragmatic process aimed at increasing consistency of approach and showing the development of the decision-making process. For that purpose, ranking scales of measurement can be helpful in real life, and sometimes it is informative to see how the ranks stack up to help generate meaningful discussions and deliberations. In case it helps to think about it, there are other examples of such aggregated multidimensional approaches to help guide decision-making in other spheres of life, for example the Glasgow Coma Scale[5] to assess consciousness, or the autism spectrum quotient (AQ-10) test[6] to help assess who should be referred for comprehensive assessment, or even the marking of a student's A-level English Literature examination.

You can design your own prioritization tool to fit your organizational context. You can develop one that is simpler or more complicated depending on the style of your organization. The key things are transparency of process and coherence with your commissioning principles, and a willingness to refine the process with any helpful learning with each new cycle.

'Within' and 'across' programme considerations

The criteria used in the tool and its underpinning principles can be applied when considering alternatives *within* a programme and *across* programmes.

Within-programme considerations mean that new proposals are considered within the respective budget for their relevant programme area (service area), for example physiotherapy, falls prevention, and orthopaedic surgery could be considered within an overall musculoskeletal care budget. Any proposal for new resources is initially screened within this programme context, and if it remains a priority for implementation in that pathway, solutions for funding can be sought within that pathway first. Only in exceptional cases would it then be assessed against a wider pool of competing priorities from all other pathways. This is akin to improving the technical efficiency of the programme budgets.

Across-programme choices refer to the consideration given to the overall distribution of resources across the many programmes of care needed for the population e.g. mental health, paediatrics, musculoskeletal, cancer care, and so on. This is akin to improving the allocative efficiency of the overall

budget for commissioning. Potentially, this overview approach to allocation could also be used to consider (or at least take stock of) the relative
allocations across different delivery settings such as urgent care, primary
care, hospital-based care, and wider community services, etc.

Such a tool can thus assist in a range of resource scenarios by helping to
make the risks, benefits, and opportunity costs of alternatives clearer for
decision-making.

Overview of the main stages of decision-making about investments and disinvestments

At this point in the chapter, you may feel you have some pieces of the jigsaw
puzzle for a prioritization process but not the overall picture yet. To help
make sense of how all this fits together, there follows an overview of the
main stages of the decision-making process for investments and disinvestments. The following stages of consideration are relevant for scenarios
when an unallocated budget is available for investing in services and new
pressures have been put forward against this fund. The principles are relevant for both within- and across-programme considerations. The scenario
of working with reduced overall resources is described later.

Screening the proposals. Each proposal is screened within their care programme context to assess whether it is an important component for that
pathway to include. Unsafe procedures, interventions with no active effectiveness, interventions that are less cost-effective than current interventions
(all other things being equal) would not pass beyond this stage. The most
relevant group to do the initial screening depends on the item. For most
items, an in-house multidisciplinary team with knowledge of the relevant
care programme could do this screening. For some items, the opinion of a
wider clinical network might need to be sought. (The criteria from a prioritization tool could be used to assist this screening stage.)

Prioritization panel stage. The bulk of the prioritization work is done at
this stage. Typically the merits of each proposal are considered by a multidisciplinary group or 'prioritization panel', using a prioritization tool to assist the information sifting as necessary. It involves the 'reality checking'
of results, understanding any seemingly aberrant results, and making any
further necessary enquiries. If there have been any unexpectedly high or
low scoring results, the learning behind why that is so is often informative

too. For example, an item taken for granted as having high priority, perhaps a mandatory item, might not actually score highly compared to other competing needs on such scrutiny, or perhaps a less high profile service area may score more highly than expected. All this will need to be taken into account in the weighing up. At the very least, a consistent application of a tool to aid prioritization provides another perspective on the relative priority of proposals. This stage can take several sessions in practice. The output of such deliberations would be a short narrative summary of the main benefits and risks of each proposal, and a ranked list of proposals. The panel is then in a position to produce a list of recommendations to present to the board (or other delegated decision-making body).

Decision-making stage. Typically an executive committee (or another explicitly delegated subgroup of the board) can formally make decisions about which benefits and risks to take, and ratifies this. In some organizations this may be the board itself. Ultimately the accountability is with the board.

Working with reduced overall resources

In a scenario of reduced overall resources, the tool and its criteria can still be used to inform decision-making deliberations. The contextual information gathered from the prioritization matrix will be useful, and a thorough understanding of the local care pathways and patient flows is crucial. Services and interventions are considered within their respective programme budget. A number of multidisciplinary teams may be involved in reviewing the relevant pathways (perhaps those where outcomes or value for money seems to be at variance with similar populations from comparative data and needs further scrutiny). Essential components for safety and quality remain. As part of this process, if proposals to refashion parts of the pathway to achieve better value come to light, they can be explored. Anything that has already been superceded by existing services, duplicated, or of lower clinical priority without affecting safety is examined further for possible disinvestment or pausing. The prioritization panel and decision-making stage already mentioned remain very pertinent. These are usually some of the most difficult decisions in commissioning and arguably one where having a coherent priority setting framework in place is even more important than usual.

Practical things for priority setting scenarios

On a practical process level, Box 10.2 summarizes key things to have in place to assist your prioritization processes.

Other uses of the matrix criteria

The criteria from a prioritization tool can also be used:

- to help commissioners, or commissioners and providers working together, to develop more robust and relevant proposals for services.
- to help make sense of the benefits and risks of *existing* services.

For completeness, the full 'matrix' tool, with prompts and guidance that the criteria in Table 10.1 were drawn from, is shown in Table 10.2.

Mandatory items and 'in-year' requests

There are two further practical issues to be aware of at this point, as they are quite commonly encountered in the commissioning for populations.

Mandatory items

These are instructions to health service commissioning organizations from external authorities to fund specific services. In the English system, examples of such directives include technology appraisal guidance from NICE (National Institute for Health and Care Excellence) pertaining to NHS commissioners, or the mandatory services that local authority public health departments need to commission.[7,8] Even if it is a 'must do' it is still useful to consider such items against prioritization tool criteria to allow the commissioner to see the risk and benefits of the proposed action, as well as being aware of the consequences if not followed through.

Box 10.2 **Practical things to have in place for priority setting scenarios**

- **Clarity about strategic objectives.** Overall aims should be clear. This is important for all types of resource situations.
- **Ethical framework for commissioning (or priority setting)** to frame decision-making in an ethical framework in the attempt to achieve strategic objectives (see Box 10.3 for an example).
- **Clarity about the role of the advisory group making the recommendations** e.g. a prioritization panel or equivalent function. This is to assess the merits of each proposal. The core panel should be multidisciplinary to include all relevant commissioning perspectives, for example commissioning overview, information and contracting, population health gain, finance, project management, and administrative support. Lay perspectives should also be considered, particularly for the development of the tool if there is a meaningful way to incorporate this. This advisory panel can also draw from others as appropriate e.g. clinical leaders, medicines management advice, communications support, wider geographical clinical networks, and specialized commissioning advice.
- **Clarity about what is the accountable decision-making body** e.g. the board or a delegated subgroup, to ratify decisions about investments and disinvestments and take ultimate responsibility.
- **A common format to gather relevant information.** Proposals that reach the prioritization stage need to provide information in an accessible format so that it can be scored with ease.
- **Prioritization tool/ 'matrix' in paper or electronic format** to assist with some initial ranking (for example, Table 10.2).
- **A number of sense-checking stages** as part of the process. For example as part of the recommendation-making stages and ratification stage to allow risks, benefits, and opportunity costs of recommendations to be meaningful.
- **Timetable or schedule** to meet, score, discuss, make recommendations, and decide (ratify decisions).

'In-year' requests for funding

Most commissioning organizations will conduct an annual review of their investments or disinvestments for the year ahead. Generically this process is referred to as the annual commissioning round. Potential investments (or disinvestments) can then be considered as part of the same overall process so that comparisons and decisions can be made. In reality there will occasionally be proposals to consider outside of this annual process. These 'in-year' funding requests typically refer to proposals for service developments or re-designs that seek funding outside of the annual commissioning round considerations. It is useful for commissioners to consider how they would handle such eventualities beforehand, so these in-year requests for funding are dealt with consistently. A practical approach taken in these situations has been that such in-year developments should only be approved outside of the annual commissioning round in exceptional circumstances, otherwise it undermines the wider commissioning round decision-making process and masks opportunity costs. Such exceptions should be rare, e.g. truly exceptional clinical benefits, or a large-scale incident. There is a wider practical literature on the topic and Austin et al. examine this area of practice in detail if needed.[9]

Guiding principles for priority setting: An ethical framework

The chapter has so far looked at the more visible aspects of the prioritization process (tool and practicalities). It is now time to remind ourselves that one of the basic elements of a coherent prioritization approach is the set of guiding principles that a commissioning organization decides to use to steer its overall approach, sometimes referred to as an ethical framework for priority setting.

In general, a framework would acknowledge the commissioning context with its finite resources, cover the main factors that the organization takes into account in its decision-making for the population and individuals within it, and should be coherent with any prioritization tool that the organization might use. In addition, and just as importantly, it can be used to guide decision-making in situations where a full blown prioritization process is not needed but the principles are. An example framework is shown in Box 10.3.

Box 10.3 **Example of an ethical framework for priority setting**

This framework sets out the overarching principles and factors that will be taken into account for commissioning decisions. It applies to all types of funding decisions that the organization undertakes, whether with respect to the annual commissioning round, service developments, or individual funding request situations.

The organization has responsibilities to:

(i) Ensure that the population served has access to a comprehensive range of quality health services secured from resources available.

(ii) Improve the health and wellbeing of the population, and to reduce inequalities in access and outcomes of services through our commissioning and by working with others where appropriate.

To do this [*name of organization*] has to use its available resources responsibly, and this may involve making difficult choices at times. A framework of principles is used to assist in this process. Priorities will be guided by the following:

- **National and local targets** that are based upon identified needs and demographics.
- **Health needs** for which effective interventions exist, and that offer the greatest benefit for our population. In improving health outcomes we will take into account measures of mortality, morbidity, and patient experience and any validated economic measures.
- **Equity** based on assessed need, which at times may result in differential distribution of resources.
- **Earlier interventions** and preventive measures with proven effectiveness and cost-effectiveness.

Account will also be taken of:

- **Disinvestment and investment opportunities.** Commissioned services will be continually reviewed within our overall plan so that resources can be re-invested more appropriately if needed.

- **Patient and carer experience.** Services should deliver standards and outcomes that are meaningful to patients and carers. We will seek to engage the views of patients and carers in developing the prioritization process.
- **Innovation.** We will encourage innovations that can provide evidence of improved outcomes, and can demonstrate how new ways of working can positively affect other services within and beyond health services.
- **Resources.** We will remain within our resource limits, and this may mean that not all services that are clinically effective and cost-effective can be commissioned. On occasions we will need to balance the needs of individuals against the needs of the population as a whole in a context of finite resources.
- **Legal and statutory duties.**

Ethical dilemmas and considerations

As informed decision-making takes place in a real-life context and takes into account multiple factors, on occasions there will be conflicting imperatives at stake and some of these choices will be difficult. Now that we have a feel of the overall elements in a prioritization framework, it is useful to touch on some of the difficult considerations that may be faced in the commissioning arena. It is helpful to recognize these situations.

Clearly, a system with finite resources cannot fund everything that providers can do and choices will have to be made. Openness about the principles and factors to be taken into account, and the processes used, will help to improve consistency and to increase fairness in resource allocation. That is why a commissioning principles framework is often called an ethical framework for commissioning.

A dilemma is described by the Oxford English Dictionary[10] as, 'a situation in which a difficult choice has to be made between two or more alternatives, especially ones that are equally undesirable'. This pragmatic definition can be used to look at some dilemmas in commissioning. Such conflicts usually arise when by trying to meet one principle it has an undesirable impact on another (for example, when funding a 'must do' service there is an impact on the resources available to fund other needed services).

In this practical arena we need to accept that meaningful decision-making is not simply a reductive mechanical calculation but involves a range of relevant considerations (resulting in a decision-maker or decision-making body taking responsibility for that course of action). From practical experience, processes to demonstrate fairness often boil down to a focus on transparency, consistency of approach, and having workable processes for review, improvement, and appeals.[11] Interestingly, these observations of fair decision-making processes and 'accountability for reasonableness' are also consistent with reflections by those who have taken a more philosophical route to understanding and articulating the handling of this area of practice.[12]

This brings us back to the three core elements needed for a coherent prioritization approach described at the start of the chapter, namely guiding principles, a tool to help inform the process, and coherent decision-making processes. Hold onto those elements as they continue to apply, perhaps even more so, in situations involving difficult decisions, by providing an explicit and consistent context for decision-making.

You may be able to recall some health service commissioning dilemmas from your own practice or studies, or perhaps have heard about such issues in news reports. Some typical scenarios are described below. The list is not exhaustive. Some are true ethical dilemmas, in the sense that it involves a conflict between two different moral imperatives, others are more general conflicts that may arise during the commissioning cycle which need consideration. All involve conflicts between different requirements.

Individual versus population needs

There will be occasions when local commissioners will receive individual requests for funding interventions or services that are not routinely funded for others in the population and these requests for funding will have to be considered against the overall resources for the population. The principle of equal treatment for equal need is pertinent here, so an intervention would not be funded for the patient if it cannot be funded for other patients in similar clinical circumstances and need. So such cases would have to be considered on their merits on a clinical exceptionality basis. Clinical exceptionality would mean that the clinical picture of that individual is so different compared to the general cohort of people with the same condition that they would gain exceptional clinical benefit from the intervention compared to others in the same cohort of people.[13] If no such clinical exceptionality is evident then the request is not usually funded as this would be inconsistent with the wider population of people with similar health needs.

Overall health gain versus health inequalities

The conflict here arises when a health outcome in a population might improve overall (e.g. fewer deaths resulting from a condition), but this may also have inadvertently exacerbated existing health inequalities in access or outcomes. For example, consider a theoretical population where there has been an overall increase in survival rates from lung cancer associated with a new way of organizing services, but the gap in survival rates between the most deprived and least deprived in the population has increased. That is, the overall gain has not been evenly distributed across the population or benefited those most in need first. This was obviously not intentional and might have occurred despite efforts to organize services to address health needs equitably at the point of presentation. It may be due to incompletely understood factors earlier on in the patient's journey which have a bearing on the outcome, (for example, differences in the effectiveness of earlier health seeking interactions may still influence the outcome, despite access to services at a later stage in the disease). The effect can be subtle but persistent[14] and remains an issue that decision-makers need to be aware of and grapple with. It is thus important for commissioners to monitor this potential effect through process measures and outcome measures relevant to the services they are responsible for.

'Must dos'

These are mandatory directions for commissioners to provide certain services from the overall pot of resources, and their suggested handling has been described earlier ('mandatory items'). The associated conflict here is that such 'must dos' could bypass the usual processes for prioritization which have been set up for greater explicitness and fairness. This relative 'privileging' of some interventions and services may come at the expense of other needs that have been prioritized locally.

Unplanned calls for use of resources

The nature of such 'in-year' funding requests and their suggested handling has been described earlier. The potential conflict in these situations is that if the unplanned item is not dealt with in a consistent way then it conflicts with the fairness principle, that is all calls for new or existing funds should be part of a priority setting process, and not be able to normally bypass such a process.

Conflicts of interest

Although this type of conflict is not specific to the commissioning arena, it illustrates that conflicts can sometimes be shaped not just by the principles adopted (ethical-type conflicts), but also by how decision-making is structured. A conflict of interest may arise for example if a decision-maker has a commissioning role and is also a provider of services within the same system. Whilst both roles may be legitimate and useful in their own right (e.g. providing insights into local care pathways in the former role, and providing a service in the latter), there is at least a perceived conflict of interest. Such situations are not impossible to navigate in practice, and indeed might have been so designed to enhance clinical engagement in decision-making in the first place, but it does require thoughtful consideration of how these situations can be designed to be optimally helpful for population commissioning whilst minimizing risks of conflicts of interest. There is a wider literature on recognizing and handling such conflicts in general and within health services.[15,16]

Potential antidotes and practical approaches to dilemmas

By putting dilemmas under the spotlight at this point rather than earlier you will have a better feel for why they exist (when needs are greater than the resources available and/or conflicting imperatives), how they come to light in the commissioning processes (for example as part of the annual commissioning round deliberations, or other funding requests), and some practical ways to handle them. Not surprisingly, there are no easy answers in this fascinating area of practice. Having a coherent approach to prioritization is intended to make things fairer, but it never promised to make it easier. Being able to see the situation for what it is and acknowledging the risks is key.

Enablers of a fairer and workable approach to tackling these scenarios include:

- Transparency of factors to be taken into account (guiding principles).
- Coherent decision-making processes for priority setting in its various guises (for example, annual commissioning round decisions, unplanned requests, and individual requests for funding).
- Gaining a wide consensus for any prioritization tool and weightings used to help gather and sift through the information.
- Sense-checking stages.
- Appeals processes.
- Continual learning approach to priority setting so that processes can continue to be refined and improved. Ongoing training and development of decision-makers (including awareness of law in this area).
- Recognition and proper deliberation of the potential scenarios of conflict.

Perhaps unsurprisingly, these suggestions relate back to and hinge on having the core elements of a coherent prioritization process in place.

Round-up

The nature of decision-making when there are multiple competing demands means not everything that is effective and cost-effective is affordable. The elements described in this chapter are the key foundations to building a coherent approach to prioritization and its challenges. A prioritization approach helps to assess if resources could be used differently within the relevant care pathway, or across the overall budget for services. It is useful to develop an explicit process for making decisions about the prioritization of resources, and try to use it even if you only have a set of ethical principles and a set of criteria to assess proposals against.

Both theory and practice need to come together for workable decisions to be achieved. The prioritization panel process needs practical support to gather and assess the information available and to make recommendations.

Ideally this part of the process includes a working group with a range of perspectives including non-clinicians and clinicians. Things to avoid at this stage include decisions going straight to a board without sufficient assessment and explanation of the risks and benefits, or without a recommendation. In these circumstances, it is almost always best to send it back and get some preparatory assessment first, because key decisions not only have their own risks and benefits but also incur opportunity costs if one course of action is taken instead of another. Enjoy working in this fascinating area and remember that a good enough transparent approach is ok to start with if it is better than none at all, and you can continue to refine it as new learning evolves. You will have something very useful quite soon.

Reflection

Think of an organization you have been part of or are currently working in. As far as you can glean, is there a process for choosing between different options for investments or disinvestments?

If so, what works well and what could be improved?

If not, how would you describe how such decisions are made? And what could be improved?

References

1. NHS Eastern Cheshire Clinical Commissioning Group. Prioritisation Tool: 'The Matrix', pp. 16–18 in, Commissioning Intentions–2016/17 Principles of Service Prioritisation. January 2016. Available at: https://www.easterncheshireccg. nhs.uk/Downloads/Governing-Body/Meetings/2016-01-27/3.3%20-%20Commissioning%20Principles%20GB%20Mtg%2027%20Jan%2016%20 v5%20FINAL%20FULL.pdf
2. Sidhu K. Sandwell PCT's modified Portsmouth Scorecard. In: Priority Setting: Strategic Planning, NHS Confederation, 2008.
3. Sin J, Dudley-Southern R, Allen L. '2007/08 LDP Prioritisation process: Proforma Completion Guidance' & Guidance Notes. Greater Manchester Collaborative Commissioning Programme, 2007.
4. Porta M. *A Dictionary of Epidemiology*. Handbook sponsored by the International Epidemiological Association. Sixth edition. Oxford University Press, 2014.
5. Teasdale G, Jennet B. Assessment of coma and impaired consciousness. A practical scale. *Lancet* 1974;304;7872:81–84.

6. NICE. Autism spectrum disorder in adults: diagnosis and management. Clinical Guideline [CG 142]. Updated 2016.
7. NICE. NICE technology appraisal guidance. Available at: https://www.nice.org.uk/about/what-we-do/our-programmes/nice-guidance/nice-technology-appraisal-guidance
8. Department of Health and Social Care. Public health ring-fenced grant 2019/20 circular. Local Authority Circular LAC(DHSC)(2018)2. December 2018.
9. Austin D. Priority Setting: Managing new treatments, priority setting series report no. 2. NHS Confederation, 2008.
10. Oxford English Dictionary. Oxford University Press. Available at: https://en.oxforddictionaries.com/definition/dilemma
11. National Commissioning Board. Commissioning policy: ethical framework for priority setting and resource allocation. Reference NHSCB/CP/01. 2013.
12. Daniels N, Sabin J. The ethics of accountability in managed care reform. *Health Affairs* 1998;17(5):50–64.
13. Austin D. Priority setting: Managing individual funding requests, priority setting series report no. 3. NHS Confederation, 2008.
14. Exarchakou A, Rachet B, Belot A et al. Impact of national cancer policies on cancer survival trends and socioeconomic inequalities in England, 1996-2013: population based study. *BMJ* 2018;360:k764.
15. NHS England. Managing conflicts of interest in the NHS. Gateway reference 06419. 2017.
16. Committee on Standards in Public Life. The seven principles of public life. May 1995. Available at: https://www.gov.uk/government/publications/the-7-principles-of-public-life/the-7-principles-of-public-life--2

11

Deciding a Sensible Approach to Commissioning when Multiple Commissioners Are Involved

Occasionally, as a commissioner of services you may be involved in discussions about whether a service should be collectively commissioned or not; if so, this may be useful.

Most of the time a commissioning organization (or 'commissioner' for short) would hold a contract with each of its provider organizations ('providers') in order to secure services for the population. A health authority type commissioner would typically have a number of contracts in place spanning the breadth of hospital services, community health and mental health services, maternity care, ambulance services, general practice services, and so on. This relatively straightforward one-to-one commissioner-provider arrangement would be how the bulk of contracts between health service commissioners and providers are generally arranged in England within its 'purchaser-provider' type system for securing services for the local population.

This chapter is to help navigate when it would make sense to consider a collaborative approach to commissioning, and conversely when other models may be a better way to get the job done.

Main point to be familiar with . . .

- When it would be advantageous to commission collectively and when it would not.

Commissioning and a Population Approach to Health Services Decision-Making. Julie Sin, Oxford University Press (2020). © Oxford University Press. DOI: 10.1093/oso/9780198840732.001.0001

Multiple commissioner scenarios

On occasion, a number of commissioners might explore working together to commission collectively if there was a common purpose and the outcomes they seek from their commissioned services were the same or very similar. There are various ways this could turn out but there are two main scenarios. The key difference between them is the degree of commitment to sharing accountability and pooling funds.

Collaborative commissioning (with collaborative contracting)

In this scenario a number of commissioners work together to secure the same service collectively, for example, several healthcare commissioners (such as Clinical Commissioning Groups) might work together to commission a common service. Usually, this is considered if there is only one relevant provider in the region, it is a well-defined service, and all participating commissioners want to contract the same service to the same standards. Examples are regional ambulance services, regional medicines management services, and some specialized services. In these circumstances a 'collaborative commissioning' arrangement may be sensible. It can save duplication of effort administratively and there may be financial advantages to working together. Arrangements change from time-to-time but many nationally defined specialized health services have been commissioned along these lines in the past (2002 to 2012)[1] for these reasons. As well as securing common quality standards, the advantage of commissioning specialized services in this way is that it can smooth out the volatile nature of the financial risk associated with high cost, low volume services, which might otherwise unpredictably impact on a single small commissioner disproportionately in-year. A properly considered collaborative commissioning arrangement could share some of this financial risk across several organizations, for example when a cluster of high-cost need occurs in one area (e.g. high-cost specialist treatment for haemophilia in a family grouping), the risk can be shared out to some extent across the collaborative arrangement, rather like an insurance policy.

Key features of a collaborative commissioning arrangement are the pooling of funds to commission the service, and a single contract with the provider (usually held by a 'lead' commissioner with a number of associate commissioners, or terminology to that effect). Effective collaborative commissioning arrangements need mature understanding from all parties about the common goals, any financial risk sharing, and clarity about ultimate accountability as commissioners. A large geographical footprint involving a number of constituent populations may be covered by the arrangement.

'Collaborations of intent'

Another scenario involving multiple commissioners exists when the responsibilities for commissioning different components of a care pathway lie across several statutory organizations (for example several NHS and local authority commissioners). In this scenario, not only are there multiple commissioners involved in securing different parts of the pathway, but there may also be different accountability systems. A typical example is the collection of services for the local children's population where there are many multiagency efforts to secure a comprehensive range of services with respect to preventive care, treatment, and ongoing care. For example, the services for children could encompass school nursing, health visiting, education, youth services, primary care, paediatrics, immunizations, child and adolescent mental health services, children's social care, and so on, thus involving a number of (fundholding) commissioning organizations. Mental health services and services for older people are other classic examples of such multiagency pathways. The many commissioners involved across the 'patient journey' with such pathways need to be aware not only of their own responsibilities but also those of partner organizations, and in turn, when it might be sensible to work together (sometimes strategically, sometimes operationally). This does not necessarily involve contracting together. In some situations there might be explicitly agreed system goals among the commissioners involved but the arrangement stops short of pooling resources and having a single contract with the provider or providers (e.g. to ensure services for children with learning disability or cared-for children are more coordinated). In these cases, the arrangement is better described as a 'collaboration of intent' rather than collaborative commissioning, as there is no formal collaborative contracting or risk sharing. Such arrangements can be for a single defined population or can be relevant for more than one population footprint.

Working out what is suitable

This section will describe a short way of working out if a collaborative arrangement is suitable, or not.

The first thing to consider is whether there is sufficient clarity about the service that needs to be commissioned e.g. an ambulance service, a child and adolescent mental health service, a cancer screening service, etc. If this is not yet clear, go back and clarify. It is not relevant for deciding whether to use a collaborative commissioning approach yet.

When ready, the next stage is to work out whether a simple commissioner-provider relationship would suffice, or whether one of the collaborative approaches is suitable.

Consider the following,

- **How many commissioners** are involved? Commissioners are accountable and can make decisions about using funds for commissioned services under their remit.
- **How many providers** are involved?
- **Is there an agreed common goal or an aligned vision** across commissioners about the service to be commissioned? Or are there several different visions? If there is no common vision then a collective commissioning arrangement is not suitable.
- **Will there be pooling of funds?**
- Which will be the **accountable organization(s)**? Clarity is important whatever the arrangement.

Table 11.1 summarizes the nature of multiple commissioner arrangements in contrast to the 'simpler' single commissioner-provider arrangement. Often the simple commissioning arrangement is the most workable. When it is advantageous for commissioners to work together to 'buy' services needed for their populations, a collaborative approach can be considered. In collaborative models, all participating commissioners have an aligned vision of the service to be commissioned. The crux of the matter is then whether funds are pooled into a single contract with the provider. If the answer is yes, then there is potential for a true collaborative commissioning arrangement. If the

Table 11.1 Multiple commissioner scenarios in contrast to one-to-one commissioner-provider arrangements

Commissioner-provider arrangement	Number of commissioners involved	Number of providers involved	Examples of services commissioned in this way
A Simple commissioning relationship between commissioner and provider. *Description:* A commissioner contracts with a provider organization to provide a service. This is the simplest arrangement. Many health service contracts are commissioned this way. A commissioner may hold many of these types of contracts. This is not collective commissioning.	Single commissioner	Single provider	• *Local NHS commissioning of:* local secondary care and community services, community mental health services. • *NHS England commissioning of:* community pharmacy, dentistry, optometry, and immunization programmes. • *Local authority public health commissioning of:* school nursing, smoking cessation services, drug and alcohol services.
A **B 'Collaborative commissioning' (collaborative contracting).** *Description:* Several commissioners work together with a common goal. They agree it is best achieved through a single contract. Classically applied to services for conditions that are high cost and relatively rare, but also applicable when there is only one realistic service provider across all those commissioning. *Funding and accountability:* Funding for the service is pooled across commissioners. There is a common commissioning process usually coordinated through a 'lead commissioner' organization. Day-to-day commissioning work is conducted by the lead organization on behalf of the other associate commissioners (or equivalent names) though each organization remains ultimately accountable for their population, *Situations suitable:* • Only one or very few providers AND there are agreed common quality standards. • Or, for high cost, low volume services and financial risk sharing is important. *Limitations:* All commissioners must be happy about the common standards of provision. Not suitable when each commissioner actually wants a bespoke service.	Multiple commissioners	Single provider, or a limited number of providers	• Regional commissioning of ambulance services • Components of population screening programmes where there are a limited number of providers e.g. laboratory services • Specialized services have been commissioned in this manner in the past (these are nationally defined) e.g. paediatric cardiology, neonatology, genetics, paediatric rheumatology. • A sub-regional 'medicines management team'.

(Continued)

Table 11.1 (Continued)

Commissioner-provider arrangement	Number of commissioners involved	Number of providers involved	Examples of services commissioned in this way
C 'Collaboration of intent' *Description:* There is an explicitly agreed aligned vision across multiple commissioners but there remain many separate commissioning processes. *Funding and accountability:* Funds are not pooled and there is no common commissioning process (contractually). Each organization remains ultimately accountable for their population. *Situations suitable:* When several commissioners wish to work together towards a common goal, but each commissioner wishes to retain direct commissioning of their own services and does not wish to pool funds. *Limitations:* There is no contractual leverage over partner commissioners to deliver the common vision. Have to trust partners to deliver the joint vision in this way.	Multiple commissioners	Multiple providers usually, but could be a very comprehensive single provider	Many multiagency efforts are organized or aspire to work in this manner. For example, the organizations on a multiagency board such as a Health and Wellbeing Board may wish to align their commissioning strategies for a particular cohort of people or condition-specific pathways such as the frail elderly, children with learning disabilities, or mental health pathways. Potentially the commissioning of services from an integrated provider (e.g. an ICP[3]) is a collaboration of intent type arrangement (albeit involving a single provider rather than several providers).

answer is no, then the arrangement is probably a 'collaboration of intent'. Figure 11.1 is a flowchart to assist this. Choose carefully because using a 'collaborative commissioning' arrangement when it is actually a 'collaboration of intent' in spirit can be difficult to manage and might not be sustainable.

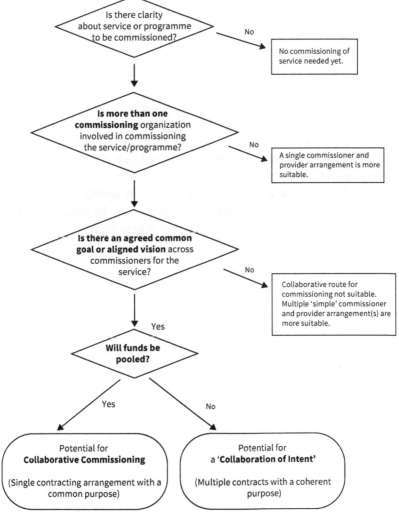

Figure 11.1 Flowchart to help assess whether a collaborative commissioning approach is suitable.

Adapted from Cheshire East Public Health, Cheshire East Council (2014). The Annual Report of the Director of Public Health 2013–2014. Available at: https://www.cheshireeast.gov.uk/ pdf/council-and-democracy/health-and-wellbeing-board/annual-public-health- report-2014-final.pdf

Don't trip up on the terminology

The generic term 'joint commissioning' is often used non-specifically. Often it may not refer to an actual collaborative commissioning with contracting relationship, but actually more akin to a 'collaboration of intent', i.e. no money or accountability is actually pooled but there may be an agreement to work together more closely. If the term is used non-specifically, it is open to different interpretations of what is actually intended, so it is best avoided if not defined. From experience, it is very rare for the term to be used to actually mean true collaborative commissioning with contracting. So it is better to just be clear about whether we are actually exploring a collaboration of intent, or a true collaborative contracting arrangement, or whether it is none of these, just an exploratory discussion about how best for things to work together at an operational or strategic level without any change to the commissioning arrangements.

Hybrids of the arrangements in Table 11.1 (A, B, and C) can sometimes occur, though often these arrangements may actually be more effective in one of the described models but have evolved or have been set up in another model for other reasons.

Summary

You now have a way of thinking about collaboration from a commissioning point of view. Through this perspective the distinguishing differences in accountability and the degree of financial and reputational risk sharing become explicit. The more heterogeneous collaboration of intent arrangements can be seen more clearly for what they have to offer and what they cannot.

An understanding of these basic scenarios helps to be more explicit about the nature of the financial, reputational, and clinical risk sharing (or to establish that there is little or no sharing of these elements). It also helps to establish who holds the ring on decision-making for what, which is important for realistic collaboration and joint problem-solving.

Reflection

Think of the ambulance services for your area. Do they serve a wider area as well?

As far as you understand, do they aim for the same standards of service for all areas covered by them? Do you think ambulance services are suitable for a collaborative commissioning arrangement across the area's commissioners?

How would this be affected if different areas demanded different standards? What type of commissioner-provider arrangement would be better then?

References

1. National Audit Office. A review of the role and costs of clinical commissioning groups. HC 1783, NAO, December 2018. Available at: https://www.nao.org.uk/wp-content/uploads/2018/12/Review-of-the-role-and-costs-of-clinical-commissioning-groups.pdf
2. Cheshire East Public Health. Looking to the future: the health and wellbeing of children and young people in Cheshire East: The Annual Report of the Director of Public Health 2013–2014, chapter 10, p. 100, 2014. Available at: https://www.cheshireeast.gov.uk/pdf/council-and-democracy/health-and-wellbeing-board/annual-public-health-report-2014-final.pdf
3. NHS England. The NHS Long Term Plan. January 2019. Available at: https://www.longtermplan.nhs.uk/wp-content/uploads/2019/01/nhs-long-term-plan-june-2019.pdf

12

Recognizing Whether You Are in Simple, Complicated, or Complex Problem Territory

This chapter invites you to zoom out a little to describe a useful vantage point to have in your toolkit for making sense of things. It is a succinct stop for interest to take a look at the concept of complex situations as they are an inherent aspect of working in health systems. Part of being effective relies on understanding the context you are operating in and a particular aspect of this relates to recognizing that different tasks and problems come with different levels of complexity. Recognizing this is an important first step in considering more suitable ways for handling the more complex problems, and hopefully reduces the chances of being wrong-footed in these situations. The important thing is to be able to recognize the situations when they are in front of you.

Essentially, a complex problem cannot be 'fixed' in a simple sense with a single solution or a defined set of activities because there are many interactions both known and unknown contributing to the situation and its evolution. However, progress can be made and if you could look back from a point in the future, you may realize how you have helped to move things on. The tools for making sense of such tasks and dealing with them more effectively might lie in having a way of thinking about the matter and including an adaptive approach.[1,2]

Main point to be familiar with ...

- Spotting the level of complexity of the job or challenge in front of you, by being able to work out what type of problem you are dealing with.

Commissioning and a Population Approach to Health Services Decision-Making. Julie Sin, Oxford University Press (2020). © Oxford University Press. DOI: 10.1093/oso/9780198840732.001.0001

Simple, complicated, and complex problems

There is an extensive wider interdisciplinary literature on the nature of complexity from many angles (e.g. the physical sciences, social sciences, and management theory) if needed and that backdrop is acknowledged. For practical purposes, the topic will be treated here as a concise but important orientation to help spot these situations in health systems practice.

The basic concept is that problems and tasks vary in their degree of complexity so methods that are suitable for tackling simple problems may not be effective in complex situations, and acknowledgement of this is the important first step in finding a more effective strategy for complex problems.

The concept of complex systems (also referred to as complexity, complexity theory, or complex adaptive systems among other related terms) that has emerged from the social policy and management arena is also pertinent for many issues in health services.[3,4,5] Indeed the importance of acknowledging complexity in health services has been noted and continues to be explored in the health literature on practice and research.[6,7,8]

For orientation, the description of problems as simple, complicated, or complex by Glouberman and Zimmerman is useful.[2] Table 12.1 illustrates the features of simple, complicated, or complex problems.

With simple tasks or problems, the components needed and what needs to be done to are easy to define, and the results are replicable. Examples in the healthcare setting include:

- administering a tetanus vaccination;
- taking a blood pressure reading;
- conducting an abdominal or neurological examination;
- diagnosing an inguinal hernia;
- calculating the total cost of 15 procedures at £1,600 per procedure.

Complicated problems involve more coordination and expertise than a simple problem but it is still possible to map out the steps needed to achieve it. There are more extraneous factors at play but outcomes still have a degree of certainty. For example:

- implementing an influenza vaccination programme for 0 to 4 year olds;
- controlling an outbreak of norovirus in three related hospitals;

Table 12.1 Distinctions between simple, complicated, and complex problems

Simple Problems	Complicated Problems	Complex Problems
e.g. baking a cake, making a cup of tea	e.g. sending a rocket to the moon	e.g. raising a child
A method or recipe is used	Rigid protocols and formulae needed	Rigid protocols have limited application or are counter-productive
Easy to replicate	Sending one rocket increases confidence of success of the next	Raising one child provides experience but there is no guarantee of success with another
No particular expertise required though experience increases success rate	Expertise from a variety of fields is needed	Expertise can help but is not essential or sufficient Understanding relationships between factors is key
Very high degree of good results every time	High degree of certainty of outcome	Uncertainty of outcome remains
Standardized product produced	Rockets are similar in critical ways	Every child is unique and must be understood as an individual
Component parts and the order they are used can easily be specified	Experts can specify a list of the parts and how they are coordinated	Cannot separate the parts from the whole
Known factors involved	Multiple knowable factors involved	Unknown factors involved
Optimistic approach to problem possible	Optimistic approach to problem possible	Optimistic approach to problem possible

(Source: Data from Glouberman and Zimmerman[2])

- setting up a musculoskeletal triage service to prioritize need and capacity;
- setting up a diabetic retinopathy screening service;
- setting up a hospital information system.

With complex problems there are many factors at play, some of which are as yet unknown and may never be known, as is the full extent of the interactions of factors with each other. Outcomes are therefore difficult to predict. This domain is akin to many natural systems, for example in the geological or biological sphere in which the exact prediction of events is difficult. The 'right answer' to such a problem is elusive and supporting data is usually incomplete. Indeed with even more complex scenarios, even agreement on what the problem is may not be defined, and there may be a divergence of values.[4] In addition, not only might the nature of the problem be incompletely understood but it may also be changing. A defined business plan in this situation has limited effect on the problem compared with its effectiveness in the simpler scenarios. For example:

- reducing the gap in life expectancy between the best off one-fifth of population and the worst off one-fifth in a city region;
- reducing incidence of mental health conditions in 5–19 year olds;
- looking after individuals with complex health and care needs to improve independence.

You can glean from the descriptions above that 'simple' planning, or a more complicated command and control approach with defined outcomes will have limited effect in a complex scenario where the outcome can only be influenced and is uncertain. Many aspects of running a health system to improve population health are akin to the complex scenario, where often desired health outcomes are the culmination of many earlier interacting factors where one can only try to influence but has no overall direct control over outcomes.

Tips for handling complex tasks

There is clearly no shortage of complex problems in real life. The question is then, what might be helpful when working with these issues. Not surprisingly, this is an area where much empirical evidence on the topic has yet to be gathered, though the conceptual level research about complexity offers general insights. The overall picture points to striking a more adaptive balance between the approach of enabling solutions from the resources and situation available, and the administrative approaches more traditionally taken for handling tasks.[5,6,9,10,11]

Acknowledgement of when we are in complex territory rather than a more simple problem territory is a first step. As there is no ultimate control in this situation one can only create the conditions for desired outcomes as far as one can. To an extent one has to allow matters to emerge within this environment and nurture those that are desirable and encourage their success. By definition, there are no simple solutions for complex problems, as any seasoned health service practitioner will know. That is not to say that there are no fruitful enabling actions that can be taken in these situations. Often the long view is helpful.

A nuanced difference between the handling of complexity in natural scenarios (compared to business management scenarios) is that there may have to be even more reliance on overall principles and the agility to spot and nurture helpful opportunities, as there is often less ability to directly control factors such as the composition of the 'customer base' and the 'range of products' offered.

The handling of complexity has usually been explored in the literature from an organizational or aggregated level perspective rather than from an individual practitioner level of contribution. Specific insights for consideration have included setting minimum specifications,[6] stakeholder involvement to improve understanding of problems, ability to work across agencies, and supporting debates on appropriate accountabilities.[4] Taking this a step further, one might also wonder what might be individual level interactions that could contribute to this end and to complement the organizational level insights? i.e. what one can contribute to help that happen (what can *I* do?). It is relevant to consider this more 'bottom-up' approach as well, as the activities and interactions of individual participants contribute to the overall leadership efforts of organizations.

Some principles on which to build an approach to complex tasks are offered below. As the literature on this aspect of commissioning and decision-making is still evolving, the suggestions are distilled from experience of working in health services decision-making and from the general literature insights of handling complex scenarios. Almost all relate to nurturing the available capability for problem-solving and creativity.

The principles are presented as ideas to help those among us who need to make sense of, and operate in, complex territory. They can be used as prompts at an individual and organizational level. The themes are:

Be open to options, be open-minded

Recognizing enabling factors in this scenario needs a level of openness greater than that for simpler scenarios if one is to avoid being wrong-footed, or missing potentially helpful courses of actions. Addressing complex problems might benefit from different perspectives and skills that come from a variety of different disciplines and experiences, not just the ones we are most familiar with (e.g. in understanding processes of care and system issues). Continue to ask 'honest questions' about the situation and be open minded about the answers.

Nurture your networks and communications with stakeholders

This might open up support, resources, and options. It encourages pooling of knowledge and is also a means of 'sense checking' ideas in a wider context. Indirectly it may enable coordination across agencies and support debates about appropriate accountabilities.[4,5,6,10] Stakeholders can be internal or external and include those responsible for change and those affected by it.

Nurture your physical and mental resources

This goes beyond getting adequate rest and recuperation, although those things are obviously important at an individual level. A lifelong learning approach, professional development,[12] reflective practice, and undergraduate training opportunities[13] can all contribute to increasing the problem-solving resources for as yet unknown problems around the corner.

Evidence-seeking approach

Often in these complex scenarios there are gaps in the evidence about the nature of the issue let alone the potential (contributory) solutions. Consider a 'do-refine-do' type approach if it is judged ethical to do so, learning from things that go right as well as things that did not go so well. Include baseline and evaluation data on the issue. The consequences will help you get a better grip of the situation. You might also wish to use a minimum specification approach.[6]

And remember what matters

To help guide overall efforts, remember what is important and what is the picture of success (for example, better patient care, or improved health of the population).

Summary

As these are often constantly evolving natural systems you are dealing with, there might be no endpoint as such. Contributions count towards the equilibrium at that point and may have some influence on the future but results may never be resolved in a permanent sense. Accepting this as a context for some of the more complex problems might help us to use resources more effectively to help to unlock and influence some of the more complex and seemingly intractable problems.

Reflection

Think of one issue you are currently grappling with (health service related or otherwise). Is it a simple, complicated, or complex problem?

Has it been understood as such by the parties involved?

References

1. Plsek PE, Greenhalgh T. Complexity science: The challenge of complexity in health care. *BMJ* 2001;323(7313):625–628.
2. Glouberman S, Zimmerman B. Complicated and complex systems: What would successful reform of Medicare look like? Discussion Paper No. 8. Commission of the Future of Health Care in Canada. July 2002. Available at: https://www.alnap.org/system/files/content/resource/files/main/complicatedandcomplexsystems-zimmermanreport-medicare-reform.pdf
3. Rittel HWJ, Webber MM. Dilemmas in a general theory of planning. *Policy Sciences* 1973;4:155–169.
4. Head B. Wicked problems on public policy. *Public Policy* 2008;3(2):101–118.
5. Uhl-Bien M, Marion R, McKelvey B. Complexity leadership theory: Shifting leadership from the industrial age to the knowledge era. *The Leadership Quarterly* 2007;18(4):298–318.
6. Plsek PE, Wilson T. Complexity Science: Complexity, leadership, and management in healthcare organisations. *BMJ* 2001;323:746–749.
7. Braithwaite J. Changing how we think about healthcare improvement. *BMJ* 2018;361:k2014. Available at: https://www.bmj.com/content/361/bmj.k2014
8. Greenhalgh T, Papoutsi C. Studying complexity in health services research: desperately seeking an overdue paradigm shift. *BMC Medicine* 2018;16:95. Available at: https://doi.org/10.1186/s12916-018-1089-4

9. Anderson P. Complexity theory and organization science. *Organization Science* 1999;10:216–232.

10. Ford R. Complex leadership competency in health care towards framing a theory of practice. *Health Serv Manage Res* 2009;22(3):101–114.

11. Reed JE, Howe C, Doyle C, Bell D. Successful healthcare improvements from translating evidence in complex systems (SHIFT-Evidence): simple rules to guide practice and research. *International Journal for Quality in Health Care* 2019;31(3):238–244. doi: 10.1093/intqhc/mzy160

12. Fraser SW, Greenhalgh T. Coping with complexity: educating for capability. *BMJ* 2001;323(7316):799–803.

13. Cristancho S. Lessons on resilience: learning to manage complexity. *Perspect Med Educ* 2016;5:133–135.

13
Quality

Are We Up to Scratch?

One hears about the term quality a lot as a health service commissioner. It is worth taking a moment to step back and think about what it usefully refers to in practice and how it contributes to patient and population outcomes. As the language used and its context is important for communication, this chapter will look at some orientating concepts on which one can build further understanding for working on matters related to quality.

The quality arena is a big topic with many facets. This chapter takes a look at the topic from a commissioning and whole population perspective. This may be useful if you are asked for example to contribute to a 'quality board' or committee, or you may just want to understand the basic dimensions of quality and their assessment in order to facilitate day-to-day dialogue about improving care.

Main points to be familiar with ...

- In health services, the assessment of quality is a multidimensional concept.
- The role of commissioning in securing and improving healthcare quality.
- The interconnecting relationship between commissioning and delivery of care perspectives on service quality.
- How to start thinking in a multidimensional way about the quality of your health services and the ways in which as a commissioner you can contribute to that.

The practical assessment of quality makes use of and is closely related to the monitoring and evaluation aspects of the 'commissioning cycle' which have been described in Chapter 4. (This is useful to bear in mind if ever 'quality' work is presented as a standalone topic, seemingly set apart from

Commissioning and a Population Approach to Health Services Decision-Making. Julie Sin, Oxford University Press (2020). © Oxford University Press. DOI: 10.1093/oso/9780198840732.001.0001

the rest of the commissioning function). Moreover, if there is an explicit quality context to the monitoring or evaluation being undertaken, there is usually a greater expectation that the findings and its ensuing learning will be used to improve services. That may be the key practical difference between routine monitoring per se and monitoring that is explicitly understood to be part of a quality assessment process.

The scope of what is assessed under the banner of quality can be wide ranging and many different activities could be considered within a quality perspective. For example, the focus may be on a specific condition pathway or a specific cohort of people (such as breast cancer or patients with frailty), or a specific aspect of care processes (such as ambulance waiting times). Sometimes a whole organization will be under the spotlight. This chapter will offer some bearings and insights so that any specific aspects you may come across will make more sense as part of understanding the quality agenda as a whole.

Overall, any indicator used is like shining a beam of light into a very large unlit cavern. Each beam reveals a part of the cavern from a different angle. Knowledge from each beam contributes to understanding the attributes of the cavern and one has to build a picture of the 'whole' from the different views obtained.

Concept of quality

There is no single definition of quality used in healthcare so it is helpful to clarify terms when working in this arena. Indeed in day-to-day use it may simply be shorthand for 'good quality'. To assess quality however, more specific description is needed.

A simple dictionary definition of quality is, 'the standard of something as measured against something of a similar kind'.[1] This starting point infers that the assessment of quality involves measuring something against a relevant reference point or standard. In healthcare, different types of standards can be used. Normative standards[2] are set by a recognized authority (e.g. government set health service standards or professional standards). Where there are no agreed normative standards, empirical standards might be used. The latter are drawn from practice and can be used as a reference point (e.g. comparisons with the national average).

As to what is being assessed when one is looking at quality, the term can refer to many different aspects of healthcare delivery. For example, the quality of the patient-clinician interaction, or the quality of a service overall, or of a component part of a service, or the quality of the behind-the-scenes organizational processes aimed at improving the effectiveness of care. It is useful to be explicit about which aspects you or your group are looking at.

Dimensions of quality

Different aspects or dimensions of quality have been put forward in the literature to help consider healthcare quality and its assessment. Any models are of course simplifications in a sense and are offered in that full knowledge, but they can offer considered and instructive starting points for making practical progress.

A classic model is Donabedian's three dimensions of 'structure, process, and outcome' with respect to considering quality in health care.[3] Although this relates directly to the care delivery level, the general concept is useful from a commissioning perspective as well. Structure in this sense would refer to physical or administrative structures (such as buildings and governance structures) and other tangible resources (such as staffing, equipment, funding, and professional training). This is the infrastructure to support and direct the provision of care. Process relates to the procedures and activities of delivering care. For example, this might include assessing patients, diagnosing, choosing appropriate investigations and interventions, reviewing patients, and professional communications. The experience of all this from the patient perspective is clearly also important to quality assessment and can be considered as part of looking at process, or more usually as part of assessing the outcomes of care.

In general, outcomes refer to 'what actually happened to the things that we tried to address?' Outcome information usually includes information about morbidity (illness) and mortality (death) and the experiences of people using services. Information about the equity of access and outcomes of services, and efficiency (value for money) can also be considered under outcomes if not considered elsewhere. In addition, it would also be sensible to consider the experience and insights of carers, and those of staff who deliver care. This would then bring in skills and insights that people have gained through their experience as patients, carers, and staff. Altogether outcomes try to gauge effectiveness, safety of care, and acceptability of care.

Maxwell described six dimensions of healthcare quality to consider in terms of, access to services, relevance to need (whole community), effectiveness (for individuals), equity, social acceptability, and efficiency.[4] These add further practical emphasis to the purpose of assessing quality. Notably many are outcome-orientated descriptors.

To some extent, the dimensions chosen for assessing quality will also be situation specific and will depend on what is being assessed and by whom. An organization might wish to focus on certain aspects as indicators of quality. For example, the assessment of quality in the National Health Service in England refers to the components of 'effectiveness, safety, and user experience'.[5] Locally you might also have a working schema that contributes to local service quality assessment, in which case other models can be used to compare with to help check that you have included what you need. Of note, across the various descriptions of quality dimensions, the outcome-related focus is the most consistent theme.

We shall now look further at the quality function from a commissioner perspective.

Quality from a commissioner perspective

Monitoring quality is about maintaining a line of sight, its purpose is to inform decisions and actions. As a commissioner there are several things we want to do:

- we want to ensure that our commissioned services meet certain standards (e.g. clinical performance against contractual standards);
- we want assurance that there are systems in place to continuously learn from practice and improve the quality of care;
- and, if quality of care falls short of expectations, to have a process for intervening if necessary.

To address these, it is worth reflecting on the practical relationship between commissioner and provider perspectives on health service quality (where there is such a distinction in functions). As the quality of services received by service users directly relates to the care delivered by providers, the commissioner's role in quality matters will be mainly through contractual relationships and effective engagement with their providers. Such commissioning roles relate to seeking assurance about the quality of services, and mechanisms to make sure that quality of care is a fundamental focus of the provider. Providers, as the deliverers of care, have to consider the many structural and procedural opportunities for delivering and improving healthcare quality. The relationship is interconnecting, with both perspectives ultimately pursuing better patient care.

Of note is that the population of concern may differ depending on commissioner or provider perspectives. Traditionally, commissioners for geographical or resident populations as in the English health system will be concerned about outcomes for the whole of the population they are responsible for. In contrast, a provider organization (such as a hospital or a mental health trust) would primarily be concerned about a subset of that population i.e. the patients that were under their care, though that is not to say a provider could not also take a population-wide view of its community impact if it so wished.

If a commissioner were to shine a spotlight on a provider of care from a quality perspective, they would wish to see the work of delivering care, a system to assess the quality of care, and mechanisms for learning and feeding back to those involved with delivering and commissioning care. Overall, the aim is to see that there is a credible system for continuous healthcare improvement.

Not surprisingly, much of the healthcare improvement literature is written with the provider perspective in mind, so one may need to read 'through' this to glean the close interconnections with commissioning processes. Do not let this deter you if you are working from a commissioning perspective, if nothing else you will have gained a wider perspective of the challenges from a provider perspective and it will help with dialogue. There is a wealth of literature on the multidimensional topic of healthcare quality drawing from business management, behavioural sciences, sociology, evaluation methodology, and complex systems, as well as from general healthcare management. For those whose work emanates primarily from a quality vantage point (whether from a provider or commissioning perspective) you may wish to explore particular arguments and initiatives further once you have your initial bearings.

Commissioner and provider processes for dealing with quality

Whilst some considerations will lie more in the realm of the provider or the commissioner it is useful to be able to consider both sides of this quality agenda together, as making sense of the connections is important for practice.

Table 13.1 illustrates a range of inputs, activities, and outcomes relating to maintaining and improving healthcare quality from the commissioning and provider perspectives. It may be useful for taking an overview, whatever the elements you choose to capture within your assessment of quality.

The table shows a collection of activities that aim to directly or indirectly improve the quality of care. Structural and process type elements are presented together as a group of facilitating inputs and activities. In practice there will also be interactions between the different components and across the commissioner and provider relationship, and that is acknowledged. The table is illustrative of the breadth of consideration and opportunities to take into account when trying to understand a healthcare quality situation and thinking about what needs to happen. Outcomes are shown as spanning both columns as they are pertinent to both commissioner and provider viewpoints.

Quality improvement is seen as pertinent to the healthcare system whether contributions originate from a commissioner perspective (with responsibility for securing services) or provider perspective (with responsibility for delivering the service). Though there may be differences in emphasis and in the tasks undertaken, both parts need to communicate effectively with each other, whatever the health service structures of the day. Commissioners need assurance that providers' structures and processes are in place to deliver a quality service. Intermediate endpoints and overall outcome information provide important feedback to this effort.

It is important to remember at this juncture that the evidence-based, or evidence-seeking approach applies to all efforts to improve healthcare quality. That means systems and procedures are also considered to be amenable to improvement with further learning, so it would also be reasonable to review the effectiveness of activities intended to help improve quality of care, such as guidelines and incentive schemes from time to time for their effectiveness and continue to improve those approaches.[17,18]

Further vantage points for the commissioner

We will now touch upon some practical points from the commissioning perspective to help make sense of discussions in this area. The first two are

Table 13.1 Commissioning and provider perspectives: components relating to healthcare quality

	From a commissioning perspective	From a provider perspective
Structural and procedural inputs and activities	**Governance and leadership** Quality functions of boards (or delegated equivalent) to seek assurance about the quality of care from commissioned services. **Contractual mechanisms between commissioners and providers:** • Contracts to specify minimum standards of services (locally or nationally set standards); • Contract review meetings, and mechanisms to raise queries and intervene if necessary; • Incentive schemes for quality improvement e.g. QOF,[6] CQUINs.[7] • Safety and safeguarding assurance.[8] **Mechanisms for reviewing and learning from wider intelligence about quality** e.g.: • (Sub)-regional intelligence about providers. • National comparisons e.g. national clinical audits,[9] 'RightCare'.[10]	**Governance and leadership** Senior accountable officer responsible for quality and health services improvement. **Physical resources** • Staff skill mix and numbers • Staff: patient ratios • Buildings, facilities • Equipment • Education and training, professional regulation and revalidation. **Administrative structures** • Health record systems • Professional communications • Information flow processes • Human resources processes. **Staff- service user interactions in the delivery of care** • 6 Cs[11] • Continuity of care[12] **Processes for continuous improvement and learning** ('clinical governance')[13] • Clinical audit[14] and participation in national audits • Evidence-based procedures and policies for delivering care.

Monitoring care delivery against agreed standards e.g. waiting times for treatment, prescribing rates of generic drugs, quality of data coding, expected outcomes.

Learning from external regulatory mechanisms e.g. inspections from regulators,[15] production of 'quality accounts' reports.[16]

Mechanisms for reviewing and learning from incidents and concerns including from serious incident reviews, complaints processes, and professional concerns.[8]

Outcomes (to inform care provision)	**Mortality and morbidity outcomes relating to effectiveness of care.** • Service specific e.g. cancer survival rates and prevention of venous thromboembolism in patients treated for hip fracture. • General e.g. falls in hospital, higher grade pressure ulcers, deaths within 30 days of hospital discharge. **Experience of people using services, carers, and staff.** **Inequalities of access or outcomes.** **Efficiency** (value for money).

offered to help dialogue and interpretation. The two that then follow bring us back to the population perspective of quality.

The part of clinical audit and clinical governance

These are two key mechanisms the provider should have in place to help continuously improve care and clinical outcomes. The commissioner will need to be conversant with these in quality discussions, for example when assessing the suitability of a provider of services, or in dialogues about systems for continuous learning. The first is clinical governance.[13] This refers to how a provider organization has a system for continuous improvement of the quality of care in place, and this includes senior accountability for clinical governance. It is as much an ethos as a system of checks and balances, and is intended to make sure that quality of care is recognized as a core part of the provider's day-to-day and overall leadership function (i.e. to be given similar prominence as financial governance is given at the board level).

Clinical audit is a key element of a clinical governance approach, to continuously improve the quality of care provided. It involves a cyclical approach of choosing a relevant topic, gathering data, reviewing against a standard, learning from the findings, implementing changes and repeating the cycle to reassess at a later date.[14] The overall aim being to improve patient outcomes with each audit cycle. This allows clinicians/staff to look more closely at the quality of their care delivery, reflect, and make changes if necessary. It is useful for looking at aspects of the clinical interaction that might not otherwise be routinely captured through routine data systems, for example examining the quality of diagnosis, choice of investigations, and choice of treatments. It is a direct way of individuals reflecting on the quality of services that they deliver. It is primarily a tool to help continuously improve quality, not a performance management tool.

Human interactions and effectiveness

For a commissioner, it is also worth bearing in mind that there will also be aspects of the human interaction in the delivery of care that are not easily measurable but may have contributed (positively or not) to the overall outcomes of care. For example compliance with a treatment regime may be influenced by clinician-patient interactions that are not routinely measurable such as the effectiveness of communication from one party to another, or differential perceptions about the balance of benefits and consequences to be gained from a health activity. These relatively unseen elements of service delivery might not be routinely measured as such, but might shape the effectiveness of care. Indeed, trying to observe the impact of such effects may be akin to trying to observe the finer points of what is happening in a 'black box' of activities that deliver care. Outside of a research approach, often the only information available about such impacts is what can be gleaned from intermediate endpoints (e.g. whether medication for high blood pressure has been tolerated, or the percentage of people with diabetes aged under 19 years with adequate blood glucose control); or from later outcomes (e.g. rates of premature deaths due to strokes or heart attacks in the population, or rates of diabetic complications in young adults) when the cumulative impacts may be observed.

The next important points bring us back to the whole population perspective.

Overall outcomes

Clearly information from both intermediate endpoints and outcomes are relevant to a commissioner for understanding how care is delivered and whether benefits have been delivered. The outcomes of a pathway are particularly important as this reflects the effectiveness of a care pathway overall. If the pathway has not reduced the burden of ill health, or reduced avoidable mortality, or there is poor patient experience relative to similar populations, then clearly attention is needed to unravel what has led to this picture. That is, the outcomes of the whole care pathway are an overall alert to areas earlier in the pathway that need attention. The importance of keeping overall outcomes in mind applies to all pathways, and particularly when the patient or carer experience involves multiple 'stops' or components of care, and these stops may involve many different providers (and many different commissioners). Mental health care pathways, children's services, and care of people with multiple-morbidities are examples that involve this type of organizational complexity.

Practical impact

As with all evaluative processes, it is the real-life impact of the learning gained from any quality assessment that is the most important point for conducting the assessment in the first place. For example, the impact as a result of an audit, or routine monitoring for quality should benefit patients and improve effectiveness of care, otherwise it would not justify the time and resources of conducting the exercise.

Is it possible to 'measure' health service quality at a population level?

'Measuring' in this sense refers to making a systematic assessment rather than just statistical measuring. As to whether it is possible to measure the quality of services at a population level, it is empirically possible to measure particular *aspects* of healthcare quality at a population level, but probably more difficult to measure with precision a quantity that captures all components of healthcare quality at a population level.

The main challenge is how to routinely separate out the aggregate effects of health services from the many other known and unknown factors and interactions that influence health outcomes. That said, estimation of the contribution of healthcare to improving health outcomes has been attempted. Such attempts have indicated that healthcare contributes about a third[19] of improvement in health, or even a half [20] of the increase in life expectancy observed in the latter half of the last century. An estimate from looking at coronary heart disease suggests that a similar proportion (just over 40%) of the decline in mortality in coronary heart disease in England and Wales from 1981 to 2000 was due to treatment type services and nearly 60% was related to reductions in population risk factors.[21] (As reduction in risk factors can also be facilitated by health service activities the contribution of health services in the latter estimate may arguably have been even higher than that estimated).

In the main, assessing quality by looking at the effectiveness of care is usually pursued through looking at care pathways of specific conditions (for example, national audits of hip fracture, stroke, and myocardial infarction care, etc.),[9] or the setting of services (e.g. primary care).[6] These viewing points into service quality tend to make use of procedural endpoints as they are more closely linked to the care received and are timelier to collate (e.g. number of eligible people who received service X in a certain timeframe). Whilst they do not give a single composite indicator of all healthcare quality in the population, such information can provide useful reference points for commissioning specific services and can complement any broader summary indicators describing the health of a population.

Summary indicators of effectiveness to reflect the entirety of health services remain sparse, for the logistical, definitional, and attribution reasons alluded to already. As a proxy, the most consistently used summary measures to indicate the overall health of a population are mortality-based statistics. For example, 'life expectancy at birth' and rates of premature deaths (deaths under 75 years of age). Life expectancy at birth is probably best considered as a historical average based on all the life span experiences of people in the population that died at that point (a particular year usually). (As such it does not 'predict' the future experience of people as it is a reflection of past population experience.) Premature death rates indicate the proportion of people who are deemed to have died prematurely (compared to a pragmatic 75 years) as a result of a health condition. It can be used to compare experience over time or across populations.

Ultimately, it is more meaningful to look at population health status as a whole rather than just at aspects that can be apportioned to health services. It is after all the health of the population as a whole that one is trying to improve through the contributions of health services. The healthcare contribution would then comprise parts of that overall picture.

Whilst direct attribution to specific factors may be more difficult to discern, an overall picture would inform about the culmination of factors contributing to health outcomes, encompassing not just the contribution of health services, but that of other services, and the effects of other known and unknown factors on health, and the interactions of all these. This can be a facilitating backdrop for local commissioning decisions and wider footprint strategic discussions.

Making sense of the population picture

If presented with a set of indicators purporting to describe the health of a population, it is helpful to understand the range of information we are looking at. Firstly to note, some of the demographic statistics will be for context setting purposes only and clearly there is no standard to achieve per se, even if an empirical reference point (such as national average) is used for comparison. Examples of such descriptors are the percentage of people aged under 19 years, the percentage of people over 75 years old, and the age-dependency ratio. The rest of the indicators will usually have a reference point and an indication of whether higher or lower is better or worse. Usually, a standard is used such as the average of similar 'peer' populations, or a national average, though sometimes a normative target to reach for is used, for example a 95% immunization rate for measles, mumps, and rubella vaccinations in children in England.

Some will be outcome measures to help us understand 'what happened to the things we tried to influence?' These might relate to a specific health condition or might reflect the interaction and culmination of many factors. Life expectancy is an example of the latter. Some will be measures of process (procedural or intermediate endpoints) and relate to things we tried to do because to the best of our knowledge, these things contribute to lessen complications, functional impairment, or premature deaths. Examples are the proportion of people receiving prophylaxis to reduce the risk of venous thromboembolism after surgery for a hip fracture, or the proportion of people with diabetes that have taken up an offer of diabetic retinopathy screening.

Standing a little further back from the healthcare process, it is useful to know the prevalence of the main risk factors for ill health in the population, where these are measurable. Then standing even further back, for making sense of the situation, it is useful to know something of the social, cultural, economic, and environmental factors that might have an influence on the population's health outcomes (where these are knowable). Examples of these distal effects would include education, income, or housing indicators. Then finally we would want to know how health is distributed across our population by geography, economics, and demographic groups. All of these vantage points on our population can contribute to the commissioner's picture of their population, provide an insight into the quality of healthcare, and can be used to inform strategic dialogue and decision-making. In practice, indicators chosen would ideally be amenable to routine collection so that repeated assessments over time are possible. You could consider collecting a 'top ten' (or so) indicators to gain a picture of your population and its health services using various vantage points as an initial backdrop to inform commissioning and multiagency discussions. (For some administrative footprints there may exist ready-made lists of indicators which if available for your population of interest can be a useful backdrop (e.g. local profiles).[22] If you need to or wished to construct your own snapshot there are many indicators you could choose. Box 13.1 makes use of the various vantage points discussed and gives examples of indicators that could be included to build up a local picture of health and healthcare quality at a population level. The examples are illustrative and not intended to be exhaustive. Inequalities of outcomes are considered throughout.

Summary

You will now have some bearings for viewing the topic of 'quality' from a commissioning perspective and an understanding of how this dovetails with the provider perspective on this topic. You will also have some bearings on how to interpret and perhaps construct a picture of population health yourself if you needed to.

Quality is a multidimensional concept. Commissioners need to be able to define what they practically wish to assess under the guise of quality. Some of that may be determined by external authorities, for example waiting times for specialist appointments and processes for reviewing serious incidents, and some can be defined locally, for example referral pathways and opening hours. A general understanding of the directly and indirectly contributing activities to improve quality across commissioning and provider perspectives will facilitate better collaborative dialogue with providers about issues of quality. In practice, you will also recognize that some of the situations you will come across in this arena will be akin to working in a complex system (Chapter 12), and it is important to continue to build on the positives.

If you are an inter-disciplinarian with leadership, sociology, and evaluative inclination, the health and healthcare quality improvement arena is for you. For anyone else who cares about better patient outcomes, this is also the area for you whether you are contributing from the provider or commissioning side of this effort.

Box 13.1 Themes for collating a local picture of health and health service quality

Population outcomes as a whole (reflecting a culmination of factors of which health service components is one).

- Life expectancy at birth.
- Healthy life expectancy at birth.
- Slope index of inequality in healthy life expectancy (in essence, the gap in healthy life expectancy between the economically best off and the worst off in the population).
- Disability-free life expectancy.

Prevalence of modifiable risk factors e.g.

- Tobacco smoking.
- Obesity.
- Smoking in pregnancy.
- % physically inactive adults.

Information reflecting wider influences on health e.g.

- Deprivation score e.g. based on index of multiple deprivation;[23]
- Teenage pregnancies;
- Statutory homelessness;
- Long-term unemployment (crude rate per 1000);
- Social isolation;
- Early life inequalities e.g. school attainment (% children receiving free school meals achieving a good level of development at end of reception year at school compared with % attained in all children);
- Air pollution.

Specific conditions and groups (reflecting a culmination of factors of which health service components are one) e.g.

Premature mortality from major health conditions (directly age-standardized rates per 100,000):

- Premature mortality for cancers, cardiovascular, respiratory, renal and liver diseases, severe mental illness.

Severe mental illness:

- Prevalence of severe mental illness.
- % of people with severe mental illness receiving physical health checks.
- Inpatient suicides among patients diagnosed with severe mental disorders.
- Suicide within 30 days of discharge with a mental disorder.

Substance misuse:

- Prevalence of substance misuse disorders.
- % completed drug treatment/alcohol treatment (% who do not re-present within six months).

Cancers:

- % presenting as emergency admissions to hospital.
- One- and five-year survival rates.

Stroke and cardiovascular disease:

- Mortality within 30 days of admission for stroke.
- Mortality within 30 days of admission for acute myocardial infarction.

Dementia:

- Prevalence of dementia.

Child health:

- Infant mortality rate.
- Immunization rates.
- Oral health in 0–5 year olds.
- Prevalence of children in local authority care.

Health services effectiveness (general) e.g.

- Patient and carer experience;
- Access to GP services, dental services, hospital care, community mental health, and accident and emergency services);
- 'Avoidable harm' (e.g. post-operative deep vein thrombosis after hip or knee replacement surgery, inpatient falls, healthcare acquired infections);

- Delayed transfers of care per 100,000 of the population;
- Emergency readmissions within 30 days of discharge.

Together such a collection would contribute insights into health status, health system delivery, ongoing direct effects on health, and the wider physical and social environment that people live in.

Reflection

The next time a news item comments on a specific part of a patient care pathway (for example about waiting times in accident and emergency departments, or delays for elective operations) consider which dimensions of quality they reflect.

Which other parts of the health system would it be useful to know more about, to gain a fuller picture about the quality of that pathway?

Which top ten indicators would you use to assess whether health in your population was improving overall, or not? Life expectancy is one that comes to mind but there may be many more to consider if the information is available.

References

1. Concise Oxford Dictionary, twelfth edition. Oxford University Press, 2011.
2. Donabedian A. Evaluating the quality of medical care. *Millbank Quarterly* 2005; 83(4):691–729.
3. Donabedian A. The quality of care: how can it be assessed? *JAMA* 1988;260(12):1743–1748.
4. Maxwell RC. Quality assessment in health. *BMJ* 1984;288:1470–1472.
5. HMSO. Health and Social Care Act 2012. Part 1, section 2, the Secretary of State's duty as to improvement in quality of services. 2012.
6. NHS Digital. Quality outcome frameworks. Updated 5 April 2019. Available at: https://digital.nhs.uk/data-and-information/data-tools-and-services/data-services/general-practice-data-hub/quality-outcomes-framework-qof
7. NHS England and NHS Improvement. Commissioning for quality and innovation (CQUIN) guidance 2019–2020. Reference 000050. March 2019. Available at: https://www.england.nhs.uk/wp-content/uploads/2019/03/CQUIN-Guidance-1920-080319.pdf

8. NHS England. Safety and Safeguarding, pp.36–39. In: NHS Standard Contract 2017/18and2018/19ServiceConditions.Updated4June2018.Availableat:https://www.england.nhs.uk/publication/nhs-standard-contract-2017-18-and-2018-19-service-conditions-full-length/
9. Healthcare Quality Improvement Partnership. The national clinical audit programme. Available at: https://www.hqip.org.uk/a-z-of-nca/#.XQowzOhKjRY
10. NHS England. What is RightCare? Available at: https://www.england.nhs.uk/rightcare/what-is-nhs-rightcare/
11. NHS Commissioning Board. Compassion in practice: nursing, midwifery and care staff—our vision and strategy. Department of Health, December 2012. Available at: https://www.england.nhs.uk/wp-content/uploads/2012/12/compassion-in-practice.pdf
12. Guthrie B, Saultz JW, Freeman GK, Haggerty JL. Continuity of care matters. *BMJ* 2008;337:a867.
13. Scally G, Donaldson LJ. Clinical governance and the drive for quality improvement in the new NHS in England. *BMJ* 1998;317:61.
14. NICE. *Principles for Best Practice in Clinical Audit*. Radcliffe Medical Press, 2002.
15. Care Quality Commission. Who we are. Updated 19 July 2017. Available at: https://www.cqc.org.uk/about-us/our-purpose-role/who-we-are
16. NHS. About quality accounts. Updated 1 February 2019. Available at: https://www.nhs.uk/using-the-nhs/about-the-nhs/quality-accounts/about-quality-accounts/
17. Scott A, Sivey P, Ait Ouakrim D, Willenberg L, Naccarella L, Furler J, Young D. The effect of financial incentives on the quality of health care provided by primary care physicians. Cochrane database of systematic reviews 2011, issue 9. Art. No.:CD008451. doi:10.1002/14651858.CD008451.pub2.
18. Marshall M, Roland M. The future of QOF in England. *BMJ* 2017;359:j4681.
19. NICE. Health inequalities and population health briefing. Local government and public health briefing. 31 October 2012. Available at: http://www.hullpublichealth.org/assets/NICE/lgb4.pdf
20. Bunker JP. The role of medical care in contributing to health improvements within societies. *Int J Epidemiol* 2001;30:1260–1263.
21. Unal B, Critchley JA, Capewell S. Explaining the decline in coronary heart disease mortality in England and Wales between 1981 and 2000. *Circulation* 2004;109:1101–1107.
22. Public Health England. Local authority health profiles. Available at: https://fingertips.phe.org.uk/profile/health-profiles
23. Department for Communities and Local Government. The English indices of deprivation. Crown copyright, September 2015.

14

What Can a Commissioner Do About Health Inequalities?

It is now time to look specifically at the topic of health inequalities from the vantage point of health services commissioning. This is an important topic in commissioning health services for populations. It comes at this juncture of the book, not because it is less pertinent, but because it is even better to recognize and make sense of what commissioners can contribute after some appreciation of commissioning practice in general.

Decision-making should be cognizant of inequalities in health outcomes within a population, and the practice of commissioning should do what is within its gift to reduce them and certainly try to avoid aggravating them. This chapter considers the wider health inequality context in which health services are commissioned, and also the tangible contributions to reducing these inequalities that commissioners can make either directly or indirectly through their role in securing services for the population. As with other core vantage points of a population approach to health services decision-making, this topic permeates many practical aspects of the commissioning function.

Main points to be familiar with ...

- The types of contributions commissioners can make to address health inequities.
- Both overall health outcomes AND the impact on health inequities matter.
- Starting early is important for health service effectiveness.

Commissioning and a Population Approach to Health Services Decision-Making. Julie Sin, Oxford University Press (2020). © Oxford University Press. DOI: 10.1093/oso/9780198840732.001.0001

Working definitions of health inequalities and health inequities

The term health inequalities refers to the differences in health status or in the distribution of health determinants between different groups of people within a population, or between populations. These differences are the result of multiple factors that influence health outcomes, including biological, behavioural, social policy, and economic factors, and the interactions among them. Some of these factors are potentially amenable to change.

Although the term health inequalities is sometimes used interchangeably with health inequities, strictly speaking health inequities are generally accepted as a specific type of inequality that indicates unjustified differences in health.[1,2] That is, health inequities are systematic differences in health that could be avoided by reasonable means.[3] The term *health inequities* is thus used to refer to those variations in health within or across populations which are deemed potentially amenable to change by reasonable means, as opposed to inherent biological factors which cannot. For example, more women than men receive treatment for breast cancer, men are more likely to be treated for prostate disorders, and older people are more likely to receive care for degenerative joint disease than children, but few would argue that these differences are the direct or indirect results of inequities in health practice and policies. On the other hand, if there was a difference in the availability of immunization for children with learning disabilities compared to children in general, or there was no access to stroke care and rehabilitation for people of a particular ethnicity whilst it was available to all others in need, these would be matters of serious concern.

So health inequalities describes that the 'amounts of health' experienced are not equal, whilst the term health inequities also expresses the sentiment that the differences referred to are unjust. The latter is in line with notions of distributive justice and also echoes the population-based concept that access to services should be based on need not ability to pay.[4,5] The concept of health inequity thus explicitly acknowledges that there is a social backdrop whereby there are advantages and disadvantages in the social circumstances of individuals and populations which may have a differential bearing on later health outcomes.

The extent that social inequalities are acceptable to society at large is a much greater debate, however the addressing of health inequities is highly relevant to commissioners because systematic differences in opportunities for health are potentially reducible, have impacts on population health measures, and should not go unscrutinized in a system that espouses access to services according to need. Whilst they cannot be eliminated, they can potentially be reduced with more equitable practices and policies.

There is an immense literature describing the importance of health inequalities and inequities from many levels and angles encompassing its determinants, impacts, and policy implications. This chapter does not seek to review this literature here as it has been explored in many other places, however it does aim to provide a conduit of the relevance of health inequities to commissioning practice, and provide suggestions to help turn the focus from principles and problem definition to practical activities as part of an evidence-seeking approach. The term health inequities will be used in this chapter to refer to health inequalities where it is reasonable to assume that the inequality is potentially modifiable with different policies and practices, otherwise the term inequalities will be used.

Origins of health inequities

The road to inequalities in health outcomes starts early and is an accumulation of biological, behavioural, social, economic, and environmental factors, and the interactions among them. These factors convey health advantages and disadvantages over time and can influence and culminate in variations in health outcomes later. Advantages and disadvantages can arise from the differential experiences in the prevalence of lifestyle risk factors, socioeconomic circumstances, access to health opportunities, and the use of these health opportunities.

These conditions in the social environment that impact on health are not evenly distributed across the population and there is a social gradient in health outcomes.[3,6] The direction of the gradient being such that the more disadvantaged a person's social position, the higher the risk of poor health. The gradient is evident when looking at overall outcome measures such as life expectancy at birth across different social groups. The difference in average years of life expectancy between the least and the most deprived groups can be many years. This difference can be summarized as the 'slope index' of inequality. For example, the difference in life expectancy between the least deprived and the most deprived 10% of neighbourhoods in England and Wales 2015–2017 was a slope index of 9.4 and 7.4 years for men and women respectively.[7] Whilst it is unrealistic to have no gradient, the aim is to have a less steep gradient.

So how do social factors manage to shape health outcomes differentially across the population? And what insights can this provide for commissioners of health services? Underlying the effects of the social determinants on health are the differences in advantages and disadvantages experienced by different groups. Across a population, social hierarchies are usually (formally or informally) grouped by wealth, power, and prestige.[8] The effects of this play out through material and social circumstances such as living conditions, the community environment, workplaces, and social position (for example related to gender, occupation, race, ethnicity, and education), and the policies and practices related to these factors. The effects of advantages and disadvantages experienced through these social determinants can directly influence health and wellbeing risks. For example, living in damp and cold housing conditions can exacerbate respiratory and cardiovascular illnesses, or occupational hazards may increase risks of respiratory diseases differentially across the social groups. Social factors might also indirectly influence the use of health opportunities, opportunities to recover from illness, and the navigation of the health system. For example there may be greater opportunity costs associated with adopting behaviours to reduce the risk of ill health, if by doing so it impinges on income and work duties; or there may be differences in the capacity to recover from illness if there is greater co-morbidity leading to a delay in recovery, or there is a less conducive home environment to recover in. The quality of care received may also depend on help-seeking behaviour and being able to navigate the healthcare system.[9,24]

In addition, the prevalence of some key lifestyle risk factors shows a social gradient. For example, tobacco smoking remains more common in disadvantaged groups.[10,11] And it seems even for lifestyle risk factors where there is little difference in prevalence, as with alcohol use, the resulting harms still fall disproportionately on disadvantaged groups.[12]

Over a 'life course', the effect of the culmination of these advantages and disadvantages and their interactions with each other on health are detected as differentials in the life expectancy at birth (and in healthy life expectancy) between different groups. This is clearly a multifactorial picture within which many sectors and services will have a role to play in influencing health inequities.

Health services as one aspect of this can contribute by reducing unwarranted differences of access to healthcare whilst keeping a firm eye on the outcomes of care. The whole population coverage of the English health system is a direct means of addressing the access issue. Whilst that is a fundamental component, there is more to the issue of addressing health inequities than universal coverage alone because of the complex culmination of factors contributing to health outcomes. Activities that address equal opportunity of access for equal need, for pre-illness intervention opportunities, and a general reduction of key lifestyle risk factors, particularly in groups with higher prevalence, are also needed to improve the distribution of health overall. Furthermore, such health benefits could arguably also help put individuals in a better (more resilient) position to tackle or offset other remaining less advantageous social circumstances which might be affecting health.

Why address them?

There are practical, moral, and statutory reasons why reducing health inequities is a core part of a health commissioning role.

The concept of fairness is probably the strongest argument for trying to reduce these inequities in health and this has broad consensus.[1,2,3,5] In the context of delivering and commissioning health services, reducing inequities aligns to the principle of equal access for equal need in a system with universal coverage. This applies to services to prevent ill health as well as treatment services.

Furthermore, there are statutory responsibilities to contribute to reducing health inequalities and their impact on health. Within the English health system it is a recognized role of the commissioning function described in the Health and Social Care Act 2012[13] and it is recognized within the standard NHS contract.[14]

Commissioning is about the art of the possible and it is possible for health services to contribute to reducing inequities. For example, we know that tobacco smoking is a significant contributor to circulatory disease and cancer incidence. We know that circulatory diseases and cancers are main contributors to premature mortality. We know there is a social gradient with tobacco smoking. We also know that smoking cessation support can be effective and cost-effective in reducing the harms of tobacco smoking in a range of population groups.[15] It is entirely reasonable to prioritize these measures as part of a population plan to improve health and reduce health inequalities, and monitor the impact of services to see if improvements around access and utilization are needed.

Addressing inequities in health may also have positive consequences for the whole population. For example, the social gradient in harms from alcohol and drug misuse is well known, with the greatest direct harms experienced by those also with the least socioeconomic resilience, however the societal effects of drug and alcohol misuse are also recognized to be borne much wider. Effective services to help those with greatest need in this case also has 'spillover' benefits for society as a whole.[16]

There are also wider professional benefits to actively addressing this agenda. It adds a purposeful challenge to health service commissioning and one that links improving outcomes with fairness. It is a meaningful common goal for multiagency collaborative work and an opportunity to foster good joint working relationships for the longer term, as well as sharing the difficult population challenges and finding creative solutions together. Above all, if things can be done differently and health inequity gradients were shallower it would benefit individuals and the population as a whole.

Commissioner roles in reducing health inequities

Clearly, reducing the impact of health inequities resulting from the interplay of social, cultural, and economic factors that accumulate over a life course requires co-operation and resolve from across many sectors and services. There are clearly roles for the health services commissioner in contributing to this overall effort.

Health services commissioning can contribute to reducing inequities in health in three main ways. Firstly, through *a focus on equitable access to services and outcomes* through their commissioned services as far as practicable. 'Access' to health services usually includes both the notions of the availability of services (for example availability of clinics for the population and opening times), and the use of services (uptake of services). The focus on equitable access is applicable across the whole range of health services, whether related to diagnosis, treatment, ongoing care, or pre-illness opportunities. Unwarranted variations in health outcomes are important to monitor not least because one is trying to reduce or at least not worsen these, but also this information might lead to new insights about different ways of addressing health inequities locally.

Secondly, commissioners can make *direct contributions to addressing wider pre-illness factors*. For example, by commissioning risk factor awareness and opportunistic advice from hospital providers as part of the provider's routine interaction with service users (e.g. the 'Making Every Contact Count' initiative), and contributions as an employer such as maintaining smoke-free premises. Depending on the commissioner it may also be in their gift to commission services to reduce lifestyle risk factors.

Thirdly, of course, through *wider multiagency work and strategic commitment* to improve local health. Health services, whether formally or informally, also have a local leadership function on health matters. This can be used to engage in dialogue with other sectors and services to shape the local environment for health. For example, through inter-sectoral ('partnership') efforts such as the local Health and Wellbeing Board structures of the English health system.[17] These are mainly collaborations of intent (see Chapter 11) rather than vehicles for commissioning services, but can raise concerns and influence local strategy.

It is helpful for commissioners to have this milieu of more distal determinants of health in mind in their decision-making, whether or not they can directly affect them. There are two main reasons for this. Firstly, even if it is not the commissioner's direct responsibility, they can still recognize the issue and advocate for change, for example by supporting other agencies that have a more direct role. Also, these are issues that shape the health of the population and commissioners should remain alert to that as part of the context that they make decisions in, just as a clinician needs to be alert to the social circumstances of their patients and their ability to engage in health opportunities effectively. That way, when opportunities arise to collaborate and ameliorate issues, they are in a better position to respond.

Although much evidence about the effectiveness of individual interventions to reduce inequities in outcomes has yet to be gathered,[16] it would be reasonable to take the following approaches as part of an evidence-based and evidence-seeking approach to reduce amenable inequities (see Box 14.1).

The commissioning perspective is taken here, though clearly both commissioner and provider aspects of the health services are interconnected.

Box 14.1 Actions in the realm of health services commissioning to help reduce inequities in health

The basics:

- Have a 'start early' mentality, as advantages and disadvantages are cumulative.
- Have in place senior organizational accountability for health inequities. (It could be part of the quality function.)
- Use an evidence-based approach to discussions and decision-making about reducing health inequities. Help add to the body of evidence of what works and what is cost-effective.

Direct contributions:

- Consider the impact on health inequities in the population as part of the annual commissioning and decision-making processes.
- Assess service specifications for the impact on health inequities (e.g. access to services, opportunities to reduce inequities in lifestyle risk factors).
- Use the contract monitoring process to gauge the impact of services on access and outcomes of services.
- Prioritize cost-effective preventive measures of those conditions that contribute most to health inequalities.[3,18]
- Secure through providers, the offering of opportunistic advice about lifestyle risk factors to people who come into contact with services (a 'making every contact count' approach[19]) and help to build an evidence-based approach for this.
- Consider a 'proportionate universalism'[3] approach in service delivery and review this for effectiveness.
- Look at outcomes by areas of deprivation and other perspectives on inequalities. Variations in access and outcomes by deprivation are some of the best described variations in health but there might be other relevant perspectives for assessing equity in your population. For example with respect to disability, mental illness, homelessness, language barriers, access to digital technology, rurality, etc.
- Adopt evidenced actions as an employer in the community e.g. smoke-free employer.

> **Collaborative roles:**
>
> - Active and purposeful collaborations to address underlying causes through multiagency commitments e.g. Health and Wellbeing Board.[17]
> - Influencing local and national policy setting to also include the impact of health inequities. For example, local multiagency partnerships exploring approaches to tobacco control, reducing alcohol harms, and obesogenic environments.

Overall impact AND the impact on health inequities matter

From a population perspective, it is not just the overall health outcomes for the population that matter, though they are important enough; the impact of interventions on existing health inequities is also important to know and attend to. As an objective of commissioning is to improve health outcomes for the population served without increasing the health inequality gradient (and preferably one wishes to decrease it), so the effectiveness of a health activity also needs to be considered in terms of its effects on existing gradients if possible, as well as in terms of its overall population effect. To illustrate, let's say we know that to the best of our knowledge a particular service is effective, for example the earlier detection and treatment of bowel cancer. As a commissioner, we would be concerned to know not only if there was a beneficial effect on reducing the rate of late-stage disease presentations, the effect on survival, and a reduction in all-cause mortality in patients with bowel cancer, but we would also like to know whether these population benefits were distributed equitably across all our patients with bowel cancer. The same principle about considering both overall population outcomes and the impact on health inequities could apply to any services (for example, with respect to stroke care, diabetes care, and interventions in mental health services).

For the avoidance of doubt, the spirit of reducing the gap in health outcomes between the best and worst experiences is essentially about 'lifting the bottom' and not about decreasing outcomes at the top. Marmot describes the approach of 'proportionate universalism', to improve outcomes for all, but for those at the bottom fastest.[3]

So, although we would like all effective activities to also contribute to reducing health inequities (or at least not worsen them), a crude approach to delivery might not achieve that in practice. The well-known description of the 'inverse care law' described by Tudor-Hart[20] suggested that there is likely to be a differential in the take-up of services with those most in need receiving the least (subsequent evidence has supported his general hypothesis). That is, in a system left to its own devices, the use of health care (generally speaking) has a tendency to be inversely proportional to need. In theory this could aggravate inequities across the care pathway from pre-illness activities as well as ill health treatment services.

Sometimes, even with the best intentions, activities may inadvertently increase inequities in access and outcomes, in which case we need to be at least alert to such effects and avoid aggravating them. For instance, an activity such as cancer screening might be taken up in a greater proportion by those already in better health than by those who might be at greater risk of developing the condition being addressed by screening.[21] Or more subtly, the intervention might be taken up in an equitable manner but successful outcomes (e.g. smoking cessation rates) are more common in less disadvantaged groups.[22] These effects do not mean that these services are not effective per se but it does mean that the effect on inequalities needs to be constantly borne in mind in service commissioning and provision. The proportionate universalism[3] approach described by Marmot and other targeted approaches are countermeasures to reduce the risk of this effect. Keeping an eye on health inequities by routinely using health inequity measures within service pathways (e.g. mental health, strokes, cancers) will provide information to commissioners and their associated providers of where to focus their efforts to reduce these adverse effects.

Some actions at a population level may be more even-handed across the social gradient, that is without worsening inequities in health, or even reduce them somewhat (for example the restriction of sales of tobacco to minors and seatbelt legislation). These may be outside the direct realm of local health service decision-making, but nonetheless it is useful to be aware of this in multiagency discussions as there may be opportunities to support awareness and implementation of these initiatives locally.

Starting early matters

For a fuller effect on equity of outcomes from health service care, tackling inequities needs to start early. The concept that starting early matters is as apt for those shaping and working within health services, as it is to those whose work lies outside the front door of health facilities, if we want to reduce inequities. There is evidence to support that reducing inequities of healthcare outcomes is not just about reducing unwarranted variation in access to health services at the point of presenting for treatment. Inequities of outcomes can exist even with little discrepancy in access to healthcare services and suggests that suboptimal pre-illness health opportunities may be contributing to the later outcome picture. That is, to achieve more equitable outcomes, actions on inequities need to start before the eventual condition is manifest. For instance, there is evidence to suggest that improved control of risk factors for ishaemic and haemorrhagic strokes would contribute to reducing inequalities in outcomes in these conditions further.[23] This would infer that reducing inequities in health is more than equal access for equal need at the point of needing treatment, reducing inequalities in outcomes is also about preventive approaches that are effective across the 'social gradient' of need. That is, for the health service commissioner (and associated organizations delivering care), the opportunities to contribute lie in enabling equitable access and utilization of pre-illness opportunities as well as to treatment and care opportunities.

Summary

By active awareness of the health inequities context, you will now have bearings about how healthcare commissioning can directly contribute to addressing health inequities through practice and policies. Many of these contributory activities are within the gift of the health services decision-maker and will be relevant to day-to-day commissioning practice.

As a commissioner you can also contribute your vantage point and knowledge to advocating and leading for reduced inequities of health outcomes in your collaborative and multiagency work. There are specific opportunities for commissioners to engage with and these have been touched upon. The overall task of addressing inequities is a continuous matter with the aim of achieving a better equilibrium rather than throwing a few things into the pot and hoping the job is completed in perpetuity.

Reflection

Think of any issue related to health you have studied or have come across in the last couple of months. Were health inequity components actively considered?
Would you approach anything differently now?

References

1. Whitehead M. The concepts and principles of equity in health. *Int J Health Serv* 1992;22:429–445.
2. WHO. Closing the gap in a generation: health equity through action on the social determinants of health. Commission on Social Determinants of Health. Final report of the commission on social determinants of health. 2008.
3. Marmot M. *Fair Society, Healthy Lives*. The Marmot Review, February 2010.
4. UK Parliament. The National Health Service Act. 1946.
5. Department of Health and Social Care. The NHS Constitution for England. Last updated 14 October 2015. Available at: https://www.gov.uk/government/publications/the-nhs-constitution-for-england/the-nhs constitution-for-england
6. Townsend P, Davidson N. *Inequalities In Health: Black Report*. Pelican Books, 1984.
7. Office for National Statistics. Health state life expectancies by national deprivation deciles, England and Wales: 2015 to 2017. 27 March 2019. Available at: https://www.ons.gov.uk/peoplepopulationandcommunity/healthandsocialcare/healthinequalities/bulletins/healthstatelifeexpectanciesbyindexofmultipledeprivationimd/2015to2017
8. Braveman P, Gruskin S. Defining equity in health. *J Epidemiol Community Health* 2002;57:254–258.
9. Public Health England. Improving health literacy to reduce inequalities. PHE gateway reference 2015329. September 2015.
10. Jha P, Peto R, Zatonski W, Boreham J, Jarvis MJ, Lopez AD. Social inequalities in male mortality, and in male mortality from smoking: Indirect estimation from national death rates in England and Wales, Poland, and North America. *Lancet* 2006;368(9533):367–370.
11. Public Health England. Health matters: stopping smoking, what works? 25 September 2018. Available at: https://www.gov.uk/government/publications/health-matters-stopping-smoking-what-works/health-matters-stopping-smoking-what-works
12. Public Health England. Harmful drinking and alcohol dependence. 21 January 2016. Available at: https://www.gov.uk/government/publications/health-matters-harmful-drinking-and-alcohol-dependence/health-matters-harmful-drinking-and-alcohol-dependence#health-inequalities-and-alcohol-dependence

13. HMSO. Health and Social Care Act 2012. Part 1, section 26, Clinical Commissioning Groups. 2012.
14. NHS England. NHS Standard Contract 2019/20, SC13: Equity of access, equality and non-discrimination. Publication approval number 249. Updated March 2019. Available at: https://www.england.nhs.uk/wp-content/uploads/2019/03/3-FL-SCs-1920-sepsis.pdf
15. NICE. Stop smoking interventions and services. NICE guideline [NG 92]. March 2018.
16. Woodward A, Kawachi I. Why reduce health inequalities? *J Epidemiol Community Health* 2000;54:923–929.
17. HMSO. Health and Social Care Act 2012. Part 5, section 194, Establishment of Health and Wellbeing Boards. 2012.
18. Masters R, Anwar E, Collins B, Cookson R Capewell S. Return on investment of public health interventions: a systematic review. *J Epidemiol Community Health* 2017;71:827–834.
19. Health Education England, NHS. Making Every Contact Count. Available at: https://www.makingeverycontactcount.co.uk/
20. Tudor Hart J. The Inverse Care Law. *Lancet* 1971;1:405–412.
21. Public Health England. Supporting the health system to reduce inequalities in screening. PHE Screening inequalities strategy, gateway reference 2017884. March 2018.
22. Smith C, Hill S, Amos A. Stop smoking inequalities: A systematic review of socioeconomic inequalities in experiences of smoking cessation interventions in the UK. Cancer Research UK, 2018.
23. Bray BD, Paley L, Hoffman A et al. Socioeconomic disparities in first stroke incidence, quality of care, and survival: a nationwide registry-based cohort study of 44 million adults in England. *Lancet Public Health* 2018;3:e185–193. Available at: https://doi.org/10.1016/S2468-2667(18)30030-6
24. Exarchakou A, Rachet B, Belot A, Maringe C, Coleman M. Impact of national cancer policies on cancer survival trends and socioeconomic inequalities in England, 1996-2013: Population based study. *BMJ* 2018;360:k764.

15
Taking Stock for the Future

Welcome to this final viewing point of the book. By now you will have completed the journey through the essential building blocks to commissioning for health gain and have encountered some bread and butter scenarios that are part of a commissioner's repertoire. You will I hope have a better sense that you will be able to look any commissioning challenge in the eye and feel you can tackle it with a positive approach and with a transparent and evidence-seeking manner. Above all, I hope you have gained a sense that the practice of health service commissioning cannot be done properly without taking a population perspective. What may masquerade as a similar endeavour may actually be a much weakened version of commissioning if checks and balances pertaining to health gain are not pro-actively built in. Furthermore, as health service costs run into tens if not hundreds of billions of pounds of public funds annually (across England) there is also a forceful ethical imperative to make the most of the health system efforts to improve the population's health, now and for the future. This is not just about public-funded health services playing their full part in delivering effective and cost-effective services (though clearly they are very important), it is also about having a population health gain approach to commissioning and health services decision-making overall.

Now that you have had chance to delve into the different vantage points offered by each topic, they could be more easily thought of as using different rooms (or areas) of a house where each room offers a different set of resources, but all add to the overall experience and enjoyment of the house. You can wander freely from room to room in any order, depending on what you need to do. You know that each room is furnished slightly differently according to its purpose and there are different facilities in each for your use. In the realm of commissioning services, being able to use your facilities flexibly and purposefully is key, as not all commissioning issues can be resolved by a linear approach alone. In this house of resources analogy, you are welcome to return to rooms freely as many times as you want in trying to get something done.

Commissioning and a Population Approach to Health Services Decision-Making. Julie Sin, Oxford University Press (2020). © Oxford University Press. DOI: 10.1093/oso/9780198840732.001.0001

Pointers and potential

As custodians of public funds to be used to improve health and health services, there is a range of questions that commissioners perpetually seek to make progress with. These range from what works, what is the general and local situation, how do we tackle quality and health inequality issues, how does the data help with all of this, how to think about difficult choices, and working with partner organizations (within health services or otherwise). These and variants of these questions for commissioners can be approached by using the vantage points in this collection to help find a way through. Within each vantage point are principles and acknowledgement of real-life practicalities to help navigate the subject. Some of the challenges will be complex in nature, in which case the approach to it can still be purposeful, but needs to be even more open to opportunities along the way.

The core concepts presented are underpinning concepts for getting started in commissioning, such as the purposeful use of information, understanding about different types of evidence, and the basic commissioning processes. These then facilitate the more overarching scenarios such as making sense of the prioritization arena, quality matters, and reducing health inequities. The benefits of being familiar with each vantage point have also been set out in the respective chapters. Beyond this it is also clear that the power of health information and evidence to help create more effective health systems is not merely the existence of such knowledge per se but also lies in the ability of the commissioner or decision-maker to use it in context and the resulting action that comes from that.

Whilst getting acquainted with the various concepts you will also have gleaned several other things. We shall gather up these reflections in turn now so that they too can assist us in the pursuit of a population health gain approach to commissioning.

You will have seen that commissioning at its best is a multidisciplinary affair incorporating several relevant expertises working together, practising in a wider socioeconomic and political context (making use of abilities in programme management, technical commissioning skills, healthcare public health, clinical and non-clinical pathway perspectives, robust governance structures, and a strategic view) inputting at all levels of commissioning activities. You may also have picked up that although commissioning for health gain includes elements that are transactionally orientated (e.g. procurement processes, payment for services, contract monitoring data collection), these are not ends in themselves. For population-based health systems, the purpose of commissioning is to ultimately improve the health of the population it serves. In that sense, the purpose of commissioning as a set of activities is not merely transactional, but it is also transformational. That is, it has the ability to change and improve things. The aim of improving health outcomes and reducing amenable health inequities through the health services decision-making is part of this.

You will also have gathered that in real-life commissioning and decision-making, whilst measurable information is a core part of the knowledge base needed, often that is not enough by itself. In practice, those planning services for a population (whatever the nomenclature of that role over time) need to be informed by three types of practical knowledge to help make sense of the health service problems they face. These are namely, evidence of what works (or where that evidence base is at), relevant statistical knowledge about the size and impact of the situation, and knowledge of the local context (local assets, pathways, stakeholder views, and generally the art of the possible). This trio of commissioning knowledge was introduced in Chapter 8, and it is useful for considering the knowledge base needed to support any discussion about commissioning.

Could a thriving culture for a population health gain approach to health decision-making happen organically, whatever the structures of the day? Whatever the answer to that might be, it is reasonable to assume that progress would be enhanced if there were active efforts to create and nurture the conditions for a population approach to thrive. Understanding more about the work of commissioning has also allowed further reflections which overlap with education and research considerations. It would be useful to consider these a little too.

Building in headroom for a population approach

A working familiarity with commissioning for health gain is part and parcel of health services problem-solving and decision-making, and as such there are overlaps with the aims of training and professional development for many types of roles where work contributes directly or supports the planning and shaping of health services. These opportunities are worthy of further recognition.

A 'build it in' approach would suggest that big picture problem-solving skills and understanding are considered within the general professional training in health services, for example as part of the health services management training and clinical training schemes, if this is not already the case. This bigger picture understanding would complement the specific learning of the particular programme (e.g. in finance, operational management, clinical specialties, nursing, pharmacy, information management, etc.) and would provide another layer to the problem-solving skill set gained. For example, those who aim to practise in a clinical setting (e.g. in nursing, medical, or therapy disciplines) would still need a big picture understanding of the conditions they come across and how services are organized to facilitate that care, and someone focusing on the management of services would need to see a service as part of a wider set of provisions for a population and all the interdisciplinary links.

A 'build it in' approach would also suggest recognizing the value of big picture principles at earlier stages of professional education too, for example as an option on undergraduate courses with a health services interest (clinical and non-clinical disciplines). Being able to examine a health problem at a population level is relevant to a wide range of health service and wider management disciplines. Such learning would be an opportunity to engage with the issues of finite resource, needs-led care, equity of access and outcomes, and effective preventive approaches in a population system. These educational and training considerations should be encouraged, at least as an option, if not already in place. As with a driving theory course, such orientation would be a starting point on which one can build through more practice, and could be applied as part of undergraduate or postgraduate training as would be practicable.

If the term commissioning is not as useful at early stages of training, it could be considered as learning about the 'big picture of health systems'. As well as providing a flavour of how to approach the day-to-day challenges in health services decision-making at a population level, it would also help to build some organizational resilience to delivering this work in the future, regardless of any external structural changes.

A 'building it in' notion would also lead us to consider the practical links to and from the research sphere on issues of commissioning. Clearly efficient relationships between the aims of researchers and those of healthcare commissioners are important so that questions about improving practice can flow to colleagues in research and the learning generated from these research enquiries can be meaningfully used by those in the practical field. In reality, there are practical differences in emphasis between the knowledge-producer and knowledge-user working contexts and these must be acknowledged in the attempts to build more seamless use of knowledge for commissioning. (For example, operational timeframes for project work may differ, or the questions that need answering and those that are feasible to explore may overlap but may not be the same.) The connection between research and practice needs to be finely tuned, and the components that might help the efficiency of this two-way flow of ideas remain worthy of ongoing exploration. Some of the research in this area has recognized the commissioning context and this is to be encouraged.

Meanwhile, day-to-day decision-making challenges continue to present to commissioners and must be dealt with in a robust and transparent way. In large part this book is a pragmatic 'bottom-up' contribution for all those who find themselves having to deal with this problem-solving gap in everyday practice (whilst recognizing the work on understanding these connections continues to be advanced).

Thriving in the milieu

The external demands on health service decision-making are unlikely to diminish. We can glean from the wider literature and practical experience that 'breaking even' and cost implications are important to decision-makers. That affordability is a key matter is perhaps not surprising as it is essential to any custodian of the public purse. From practical observation, reducing perceived reputational risk can also feature as a predominant driver if not tempered by health gain dimensions. There will also be externally driven priorities to deliver. The influence of these external factors on decision-making have also been observed in the literature.[1] All these factors have to be acknowledged and reckoned with alongside health gain aims if we are to optimize health gain from this scenario. It is in this milieu that all those involved in commissioning services for the population are guardians of the population health gain approach.

So the overall aim is about optimizing health gain whilst breaking even. This is not insurmountable. A population health gain approach has to be part of the fabric of commissioning. That is, as part of the commissioning cycle stages, part of prioritization considerations, part of board level or delegated decision-making, or single executive decision-making. Despite the external factors, there are of course practical enablers an organization has control over and can put into place. Core enablers would include:

- An ethical framework for commissioning which is relevant for all levels of decision-making about resources.
- Provision of orientation to commissioning for health gain concepts for all staff involved in commissioning (purpose of commissioning; definition of 'health need'; a needs-led and evidence-seeking approach; awareness of effective preventive opportunities; care pathway considerations, etc.).
- An intra-organizational system for knowledge. It is insufficient merely to have information out there, it needs to reach those who can make use of it. As a baseline, core level evidence retrieval and critical appraisal skills should be a routine part of professional development.
- Ensuring there is a population health gain view in decision-making at strategic and day-to-day business levels.
- Consideration that everyone's role has both transactional and transformational contributions so a whole organizational approach to professional development in commissioning for health gain is needed, not just for those with higher profile decision-making roles.

***

Evolution and commissioning

Structures in health services will continue to change and evolve but the importance of a population approach to health services decision-making will remain as long as universal coverage of health services continues. In the academic knowledge sector there is a phrase K* ('K star') to denote 'knowledge whatever'.[2] To some extent this book is an attempt to prepare for an ongoing evolving world of commissioning* or 'commissioning whatever'. That is, whatever the nomenclature of the structures of the day, the fundamental purpose of commissioning is to secure services for the population served within finite resources, in a needs-led fashion, and address health inequalities in access and outcomes where possible.

I hope this book helps you to spot and make the most of your opportunities to commission for health gain in the system you work in. Enjoy using the vantage points and I hope it helps make your work be 'that bit easier and that bit clearer' as you contribute to the exciting field of health services decision-making for populations.

References

1. Williams L, Brown H. Factors influencing decisions of value in healthcare: a review of the literature. University of Birmingham, July 2014. Available at: https://www.nhsconfed.org/-/media/Confederation/Files/Publications/Documents/DOV_HSMC_Final_report_July_281.pdf
2. United Nations University. Expanding our understanding of K* (KT, KE, KTT, KMb, KB, KM, etc.) A concept paper from the K* conference, Ontario, 2012. Available at: https://assets.publishing.service.gov.uk/media/57a08a6e40f0b649740005ba/KStar_ConceptPaper_FINAL_Oct29_WEBsmaller.pdf

Glossary

Assurance: From the commissioner's perspective this refers to being confident that a provider organization has policies and activities in place to oversee and deliver quality services.

Atrial fibrillation: A common form of abnormal heart rhythm and a risk factor for stroke. It results from electrical impulses firing from different places in and around the upper chambers of the heart (the atria) in an uncoordinated way.

Attrition bias: A bias that occurs if losses to follow-up in studies occur differentially across exposure groups. It is a type of selection bias. It is a particular consideration in randomized controlled trials and in (prospective) cohort studies.

Bias: This refers to any systematic error in the research methods that leads to an incorrect estimation of the true effect. It can arise from systematic errors in the handling of data collection, analysis, interpretation, or publication of studies, leading to observation of differences that are not there or observation of no difference when there is one. Careful study design is needed to reduce bias in studies as it cannot be adjusted for in later analysis. The two main types of bias are selection bias and observation bias.

Care pathway: The main steps in the care of those with a specific clinical problem, or particular health needs. Also known as a service pathway or a patient journey. It is also a way of setting out a process of good practice to be followed.

Clinical Commissioning Group (CCG): A type of health service commissioning organization created following the Health and Social Care Act 2012. They were set up as clinically led statutory NHS bodies responsible for commissioning the bulk of health services for their respective areas.

Confounder (confounding variable): A variable that distorts the measured effect of exposure on the outcome. It can lead to observation of differences that do not exist or observation of no difference when they do exist.

Deprivation index: An indicator of relative deprivation of an area. It is commonly expressed as the percentage of neighbourhoods in a local authority area that are from the most deprived deciles or quintiles (10% or 20% respectively) of neighbourhoods in England.

Disability free life expectancy: An estimate of the number of years lived without a disabling health condition, on average for a person in a population.

Dose-response: An observed relationship between the amount of stimulus or exposure and the reaction observed.

Effectiveness: The extent to which intended benefits are achieved for the population under usual conditions of care.

Efficiency: The outputs obtained for the inputs invested (general).

Epidemiology: The study of the distribution and determinants of health-related states in populations, and the use of this learning to control health problems.

Grey literature: Reports by agencies that have not been published in peer-reviewed journals but contribute to inform practice.

Health gain: A term for the measurable improvement in the health of a population or individual as a result of a course of action.

Health and wellbeing board: A multiagency forum at a local authority geographical footprint introduced with the Health and Social Care Act 2012, to consider health and wellbeing priorities of the area and develop local strategy. Statutory members include representatives from the local authority, local NHS commissioners and Healthwatch (a statutory forum for users of health and social care) and other representatives as locally agreed.

Healthy life-expectancy at birth: An estimate of the average number of years that would be lived in 'good general health' for someone who has just been born, if the levels of good health and mortality rates at that point in time continued unchanged into the future.

Hyper-acute stroke unit: Specialist centres to manage the first 72 hours of stroke care.

Incidence rate: The number of new cases of a condition in a specified period in a population. For example expressed as the number of new cases per 1,000 or per 100,000. With age-standardized incidence, age structure in the population has been taken into account so that incidences can be compared over different geographies or time without differing age structure skewing the results.

Index of Multiple Deprivation (IMD): A composite score combining a number of socio-economic indicators to describe relative levels of deprivation across a geographical population. It provides an overall score at the small neighbourhood area (lower layer super output area) which can be used to build up a deprivation indicator for larger areas such as a local authority area.

Joint strategic needs assessment (JSNA): A locally produced publication about priority health issues and health needs produced at a local authority level to inform planning of local health and care systems.

Life expectancy: The number of years an individual of a given age is expected to live on average, if current age-specific mortality rates continue.

Lower Layer Super Output Area (LSOA): The smallest geographical areas in England and Wales where a range of population datasets are collected. They can be aggregated up to form larger areas for statistical analysis. LSOAs have a minimum of 1,000 residents.

Making Every Contact Count: An approach to making opportunistic use of the vast number of day-to-day interactions that health and other organizations have with people, in order to support people in making positive changes to physical and mental wellbeing.

Metabolic risk factors: Routine indicators of body processes that in combination increase the risk of developing cardiovascular disease and diabetes. These include high blood pressure, high blood sugar, lipid ratios, and waist–hip ratio.

Middle Super Output Areas (MSOA): Aggregations of Lower Layer Super Output Areas in England and Wales. MSOAs have a minimum of 5,000 residents.

National Institute for Health and Care Excellence (NICE): An arm's length National Health Service body providing guidance, recommendations, and sometimes directions to the health system in England.

Natural history of condition: The course a health condition takes from its discernible beginnings to its resolution (to recovery, chronic state, or death).

Needs-led approach: A manner of problem-solving or decision-making that is driven by the health needs of people rather than by the services available.

Number Needed to Treat: The average number of patients who need to receive the treatment or other intervention for one of them to obtain the positive outcome in the time specified. The closer the NNT is to 1, the more effective the treatment.

Observation bias: A type of bias arising when there are differences in obtaining information from different groups in a study, and therefore events are reported in a none comparable way. These differences in obtaining information can be related to the investigator (interviewer bias), or the study participant (recall bias).

Old age dependency ratio: A ratio of the number of older adults compared to younger adults. For example, the number of people over 65 years old for every 1,000 people aged between 16 and 64 years old.

Opportunity cost: The option(s) not pursued as a result of using the same resources for another option.

Prevalence: The proportion of people with a specific health condition in a defined population, at a specified point in time.

Selection bias: a type of bias arising from the methods of selecting individuals for a study or for analysis. A particular consideration in case-control and retrospective cohort studies as exposure and outcome have occurred when individuals are selected into the study.

Slope index of life expectancy at birth: The difference in life expectancy at birth between the experience of the best off and the worst off 10% (deciles) in a population.

Technology appraisal guidance (TAG): A specific type of instruction issued by the National Institute of Health and Care Excellence in England to the NHS about commissioning specific therapies and procedures. They are in effect directives to commission certain technologies.

Index

Tables, figures and boxes are indicated by *t*, *f* and *b* following the page number

For the benefit of digital users, indexed terms that span two pages (e.g., 52–53) may, on occasion, appear on only one of those pages.